Winning the Struggle to Be Thin

by Casey Conrad

Published by Communication Consultants
11 Kenyon Avenue
Wakefield, RI 02879

Visit our website at www.winningthestruggle.com or www.winningthestruggle.com.au.

ISBN: 0-9788024-0-3
Cover design by Ben Bolt, Mythic Design Studio
Cover photos: Denise Huffman, Kathy Turner and Rebel Whale
Printed in the United States of America

Contents

Acknowledgements

First I would like to acknowledge all the women featured in this book who unselfishly submitted their heart-felt stories in the hopes of inspiring other women to win their struggle to be thin. Without their stories the book would not have been possible.

Next, to all the Healthy Inspirations Centers who participated in the essay contest and helped to organize all the photos and paperwork. It is the Center operators that make the success stories happen!

To Barbara Daniels, mentor and friend, Marty Conrad, and Diane Sprague for all their tireless work in the editing of this book.

The staff at Healthy Inspirations Corporate, including Jean Gilligan, Bonnie Ellis, Cindy Martin and Susan Johnson. Their support was critical.

To my good friend and Australian distributor Jamie Hayes and his Aussie team, including Ellen Hayes, Chelsea McLean, Matt O'Neil, Rebel Whale and the support team at Australian Corporate.

To Ben and Jessica at Mythic Design Studio for their patience and dedication to creating a wonderful book cover design.

Finally, to the staff at Narragansett Graphics for doing a wonderful job in putting the pieces together.

Chapter 1

Understanding The Struggle

Confession #1

Are you letting life pass you by because, being as heavy as you are, you think you have nothing to look forward to? Well – that is what I have thought during many phases of my life – especially as it relates to my struggle with weight loss over the years. I am not much of a writer, but here's the story I would like to share.

My Mom told me I was a ten-pound baby at birth, so I guess it all began there. She said she ate two rows of Oreos each night before going to bed, so was that the beginning for me? Must have been all her fault that I became so heavy, right? I have to blame someone. I was chubby all through grade school and middle school, and I can remember having a mad crush on a guy named Alan, but he told my friend that he thought I was too "chubby", so that ended that love affair very quickly. But what about my terrific personality? Who gives a hoot about that!

By the time I got to high school, I was no longer titled "chubby" – now I was just plain "fat." So I began to do some mini-dieting on my own while playing the dating game through high school and college to keep up with the other girls. It was very difficult for me as I did spend a lot of time and energy thinking about food and what was going to be my next meal, so it was a real effort for me to put these thoughts aside. I used to love it when my parents would go out and leave my sister and me alone, so I could raid the refrigerator and eat junk food. I often did this because I felt depressed that my mother did not put what I thought was enough food on my plate during meals. So, I became a sneak eater and didn't eat too much in front of anyone. Who was I kidding? So, I would binge, then not eat much for a couple of days, and this seemed to keep my weight somewhat under control for those few years.

I slimmed down long enough to catch my husband, but by the time my wedding day arrived, I was already on the upswing with my weight. When I marched down the aisle, I was no slim, trim bride in my size 16 wedding dress. I blamed the fact that the dress was white rather than black for the reason I looked so heavy. It is amazing what you can talk yourself into when you are desperate and trying to look attractive. My hair looked good though! My poor husband, boy—love is blind!

The first year of marriage things were terribly comfortable, and things got progressively worse as my weight escalated. Not having much income, as my husband was still in college, our meals consisted of spaghetti and macaroni and cheese. Carbohydrates were cheap, and I didn't know how to cook much else, so the pounds began to pile on. Bread was also a staple in our household. What else could we possibly use to soak up the sauces?

So, my "real" weight loss journey began in 1972, after one year of blissful marriage. Now a full-figured 210 pounds, I decided that it was time to lose some of my excess poundage. Of course, my husband, God bless his skinny little rear (still the same weight today as 31 years ago), coaxed me along, and this gave me the hint that perhaps I was not looking too terrific to him anymore. He didn't have a clue as to how hard it was for me to give up food because he never had to. I think he was pretty disgusted with me, not so vocal, but the look in his eyes told the story. I was worried sick that I couldn't survive without ½ pound of pasta every day, but I decided to give my first real "diet" a try.

My first weight loss was a huge success Eight months of nothing but meat, eggs and water and almost 100 pounds vanished. Wow, I was gorgeous. Who needed exercise? So what that I was up all night with leg cramps. I looked so damn good, it didn't matter. I remember having size 8 shorts on and life was grand again. We were living in Florida at the time, and we decided to go home to Connecticut to visit our family and friends, and they had not seen me in a year. Were they ever shocked!

I remember on the airplane a guy sitting next to me was flirting, and even my husband was grinning. Of course, I didn't tell him how good it felt to have another man show me some attention after feeling so undesirable for so long. Good thing my husband was with me. Truthfully, I only flirted back for a moment because I felt so good that my husband was proud of the way I looked. That memory is so powerful for me that I hung onto that green, size 10, fitted dress for years.

So home to Connecticut we went. I had lots of new clothes and was getting tons of compliments, all of which was very exciting for me. Moments after arriving at my Mom's house, though, I began to take a nosedive. I came face to face with a pan of homemade brownies and all the old feelings for my love of food washed over me, almost consuming me. I felt myself losing control that first night. I had been so very deprived, but I looked so good. "I'll do better tomorrow," I said as I started to dive into the food. Sure, for an instant I thought to myself, "You look so good, don't blow it now," but all the food looked so delicious. I dove into the brownies, then the chips and then the beer to the point where I actually made myself sick that night. Of course, I justified it by telling myself, "You deserved it, you have been good for so many months. Just one night isn't going to kill you." But one night led to two, then three, and then a week and by the time we left Connecticut to go back to Florida I had gained 15 pounds in just two weeks. When I stepped on the scale to discover this, I was so disgusted with myself that I got depressed, which only led me to more eating, more "weight" pain. It disgusts me just sitting here writing about it!

Of course, back in Florida the next week turned into the next and so did the next whole year. It was a happy time for me to eat what I wanted to, and what the heck, I still had all my fat clothes, and the pressure was off. I didn't have to look good for anyone as we weren't going anywhere. I got great comfort from the food I ate, and I just didn't care how I looked or felt. My leg cramps were gone now because I was getting plenty of dairy (ice cream is a dairy, right?). But now new problems were developing. Of course, my husband's evil eye was hovering over me, but now my knees and back were giving me problems. I kept saying it will get better, but it didn't, and after about three years, I was over 200 pounds again. The time had come to get serious about another diet.

How depressing for me to even think about it. Food was my best friend. I used food when I was happy or sad or depressed and it gave me much comfort. My cooking skills had improved dramatically, and I enjoyed entertaining and having dinner parties. Nobody seemed to care that I was getting fat because everyone loved my cooking and the parties were great. Of course, no one but I was packing on the weight. I had my own private parties, too, just me and food, and this had to come to an end soon, at least this is what I kept telling myself.

I had failed at keeping my weight off from the last program, but no big deal because I knew I could do it again, and there were plenty to choose from. I must have gained my weight back because I picked the wrong diet, right? Well, that sounded about right. So, I heard about this prepackaged food program and it sounded pretty good. I decided to go for the consultation and see what it was all about. Only $60 per week to buy your prepackaged food; "I can do this," I thought to myself. I figured it was probably what the astronauts ate, so it must be good. And I felt very in control knowing that was all that I could eat, and there were no decisions to be made. It was all boxed up in portion control. Of course, nothing tasted that great, so I wasn't so anxious for my next meal.

My husband couldn't understand why I would spend so much on that type of food when I could buy healthy food for both of us from the grocery store. What did he know about diets? Nothing. That "buy healthy food" comment just didn't work for me because it gave me too many decisions and too much room to make mistakes. To me, eating 5 pounds of Bing cherries at one sitting sounded like healthy eating! Better for me to be in control and buy the prepackaged food. So, another success headed my way. The pounds were dropping very easily to the tune of 80 pounds lost in about 6 months. I even packed all my food for a week long vacation to the Bahamas. Wasn't that normal to eat my meal in my room before we went to the restaurant and then watch everyone else eat while I drank water? That was until the last night, when I decided to "reward" myself for having been so disciplined during the entire vacation; I ate and drank what I wanted to the point where I made myself sick and could barely get on the plane the next day.

Even after having fallen off the wagon, though, I looked "hot." The new me blossomed; the compliments streamed in and all those wonderful feelings returned. The feeling of accomplishment was overwhelming, and back to the thin clothes I went. Who cares that they were outdated. So what if bell bottoms were passé? I felt great, like I could conquer the world. I kept thinking to myself, "Thin tastes so good. I will never eat badly again. This is the final straw for me—I am forever thin."

I was feeling cocky as the weeks passed, and I decided to drop out of my program and go onto regular food. Surely I could do this on my own just by eating healthy. I also thought perhaps I should try some exercise seeing as I had done none. So off to the store I went with a million questions. "Isn't pasta healthy as long as I exercise? Can I eat all the fruit I want? I mean, it's healthy, right?" Quickly my feelings of being out of control returned. I thought to myself, "But I'm a success. I just lost over 80 pounds, I can't possibly fail again. I won't fail again!"

WRONG. One by one the pounds started finding their way back on me. At first I felt sad but then relaxation set in. What the heck – no pressure if you are not worried about what you eat. Who cares anyways – people like me for who I am, not my weight, right? Oh sure, I cared; but I just buried those feelings of failure once again. I knew I was still a nice person; people have to accept me the way I am. Fat people are always more jovial anyways – I guess because we eat what we want and don't worry about the consequences. Certainly I was always the life of the party, and nobody cared that I was overweight, but deep down, I did. I covered it up with lots of laughter and jokes. Nobody saw the inner turmoil that was going on within me and the disappointment in me. Not to mention the aggravation of finding something that fits for an event. Two or more hours to get ready— practically everything from the closet strewn all over the bed.

So, I was back up to 200 pounds again, and the biggest excuse ever for not dieting came and was welcomed; I was pregnant and eating for two, right? All three of my pregnancies were close, and I only gained a few pounds with each one because my own body weight was so high to begin with and I really was trying to eat healthy for the baby. I wasn't worried about my health, but felt a need to take care of myself for the unborn children. I ended up not gaining much weight from the pregnancies and actually lost some of my own body fat during these times. Needless to say, all three of my deliveries were most difficult due to my weight, but I managed to produce two healthy sons. Maybe it would have been three if I had taken better care of myself, but I try not to look back and beat myself up.

So the years fly by, no time for me – soccer games, school, laundry, owned a business—excuses, excuses, excuses. The kids loved pasta, so mom was right in there with them chowing down. Lots of fruits and vegetables in the house for the kids because I trained them from the beginning to eat properly and develop good eating habits—so they wouldn't end up like me. I would wait to tuck them in at night before I would pull out all the hidden junk food for me. I didn't let them eat it as I was worried about their teeth and their weight, so there was plenty for me. You see, I never wanted them to go through what I had dealt with my entire life; why would I ever want them to end up like me? No parent would wish the weight loss struggle on their child! Sure, I cared about them; I just didn't care enough about me. I would finish what was on their plates, too. Dad works hard, so let's not be wasteful. All the kid's friend's moms looked so good, and I felt terrible alongside of them, but not bad enough to do some- thing. I was always so tired and decided maybe Monday I would do something. Reminds me of a line from a popular song; "Monday, Monday, can't trust that day."

Next, I decided to try weekly meetings, as one night a week wasn't going to kill me. I wasn't sure where the meeting was, but they told me I would know which room to go to when I got to the building. Sure enough, I knew. A bunch of wide glides, waddling and breathing heavy as we all climbed the stairs to get to the meeting. But when I had to stand up in front of everyone and introduce myself as a "compulsive overeater," I was horrified, embarrassed and talked myself into the fact that I did not belong there, and this was not me. I am not a compulsive overeater, am I? What was I? If you have never lived inside a fat body, you cannot understand what was going on in my mind. You might call it weak, but if you do, you do NOT understand what it is like to be overweight.

My next plan was another weekly meeting. This program has been around for years and was definitely going to work for me. Weigh and measure food – that seemed pretty good so far as long as I stayed within so many points per day. Hey – French fries are only 15 points, and I would still have 10 more to go. That will work. It did – about ½ to 1 pound a week and soon enough I had lost 50 pounds—again. I often wondered, "Where does all the lost weight go?" But no need to ponder on that question too long because I was a winner—again.

Now hubby buys me a treadmill for Mother's Day. Isn't that romantic, telling me to get off my fat butt and exercise. Guess what, my treadmill made a great clothes hanger in our bedroom. It was just too much work to do it, so back to the couch. But the weekly meetings were okay. On weigh-in day, after I had lost a pound, everyone clapped, and I felt I needed a reward, as I didn't have to weigh-in for another seven days, so off I went to McDonald's for a treat. I always rewarded myself with food by saying, "After I lose so many pounds, I will treat myself to my favorite restaurant and eat what I want." Of course, I was setting myself up for failure by doing this. There are tons of other things in life besides food to reward yourself with – why not sex or something else, right? But no, I chose the food.

Next thing I knew, the kids were in their mid-teens. I can't get over how quickly life goes by, but I still wasn't going anywhere with my weight, but up. Where did all those years go? Time flies when you are having fun and out of control. I decided now I needed something for me as the kids didn't need so much of my time now. I knew I should try and get healthy, but I took a different route and was doomed. A local candy store went out of business and I decided that would be fun, so I reopened it. I had great success – Godiva Chocolates were the ultimate but acne at 44 was the pits. My husband could not figure out why the profits were so low. Hello!!! After a short time, and about 20 more pounds onto my body, I decided to sell and get out before it was too late. It was a fun adventure, but it certainly was not the direction I wanted to go.

I then took a bookkeeping job at a town recreation department which gave me a free membership to their pool. I was doing some self-dieting at that time and some swimming, but the coffee and donuts on my desk were getting the best of me. I once again reached a comfort level, and my weight reached an all-time high. Four years later, life was really passing me by, at 50 years of age my husband and I moved back to our hometown. We bought a boat, but being in a size 20 bathing suit was not so much fun. What a terrific co-captain I was. My husband asked me to hop up on the bow and tie the line, and I couldn't even get my leg over the side of the boat to get up to the bow! I felt like such a burden and was absolutely no help to my husband. How could he possibly have fun with his new toy with a "slug" like me? He should have just used me as the anchor because I felt like one around his neck. To say the least, I was mortified and knew that something had to give. I better do something soon so I can at least be more agile to help on the boat. The kids were gone now, so what excuses could I possibly have.

On a visit home from Arizona, my younger son who was a personal trainer at the time, told me that when I got up out of the chair after sitting for awhile I reminded him of his grandmother hobbling around. She has osteoporosis and is in a walker. Boy – was that like a knife going through my heart thinking my good looking son saw me as an old, unhealthy lady. But it was true, my knees hurt so bad; especially after sitting for awhile. That happens when you weight 200+ pounds again. This could not have possibly happened again, could it?

So, where does it stop? How the heck do you get off this nightmare ride? How much pain—physically, financially, spiritually and emotionally—will I allow myself to be subjected to before I find a solution, before it's too late? Can anyone help me? 57 years later and I sit here writing, planning, and hoping, but STILL overweight. Talk about feeling like time is slipping away. Have I spent too much time and energy on this—like 47 years too many; there has to be more to life than dwelling on my weight. Is there still time to do something or is it too late?

Anonymous
Stonington, CT

Can we even begin to understand the magnitude of this woman's struggle? Maybe you have a similar story? Even if your weight loss struggles haven't been as dramatic, if you have gained and lost weight more than once in your life, you can empathize with this woman and relate to the numerous and complex issues surrounding the struggle to be thin that are present before, during and after the weight loss process. Certainly every person faces a unique struggle, but you are not alone. Many stories of women who have lost weight have amazing similarities.

The most obvious is a pattern of weight gain and loss called "Yo-Yo dieting" or the "Oprah Syndrome" (after the famous talk show host Oprah Winfrey who has had a lifelong–and very public–struggle with her weight). Typically, this syndrome involves following the latest fad diet, some of which are sensible and some of which are not. Regardless of the choice of diet, many of them result in weight loss–in some cases incredible weight loss–but it's usually only temporary. Whether it was the diet that failed the dieter or the dieter that failed the diet, the end result is the same–more weight gain--and so the cycle starts all over again.

Whether it is bad knees, swollen feet, poor sleep, an aching back or shortness of breath with the slightest activity, the weight struggle is often accompanied by a struggle with physical pain or deteriorating health caused by excess weight. Unfortunately, many women admit that the physical pains caused from being overweight are often less painful than the thought of not eating their favorite foods. Many women confess that this illogical thinking contributes to the psychological conflict about losing weight.

Hear how Gretchen Williams overcame the cycle of yo-yo dieting and lost over 48 pounds.

Confession #2 on p. 103

The gain and loss of yo-yo dieting is often accompanied by a torrent of emotions surrounding weight and body image. On one hand these women want to be thinner and healthier, but find themselves battling emotional issues surrounding food, such as "when I eat I feel comforted, gratified, loved, or secure." Certainly, women who eat for emotional reasons logically know they shouldn't be reaching for ice cream simply because they have had a bad day, but for some unknown reason they can't seem to say no to certain temptations. This is particularly true during stressful times, during menstrual cycles, or any other times of feeling out of control, overwhelmed, or needing the instant gratification that food can provide. Of course, women admit to feeling disappointed in themselves when they fall off their diets. Unfortunately this disappointment, in turn, leads to an attitude of "What the heck, I've blown it now so I might as well just enjoy myself," which only exacerbates the problem physically and emotionally, recreating the same vicious cycle: overeat, gain weight, get depressed, eat because you're depressed, gain more weight, get more depressed, etc.

Learn how Frances Leiter lost 44 pounds and "ditched her cane" after winning her weight struggle

Confession #3 on p. 105

Another often cited psychological aspect of being overweight is the amount of time each day spent thinking about ones' weight in some way or another. Taking extra time each morning trying to find something to wear that either creates a slimmer look or at least hides the excess weight; thinking about what to eat for lunch or dinner; ordering at a restaurant and being concerned about what the waiter will think if you order something fattening; being invited to a function and having to be concerned about if the seats will be comfortable, large enough—or even collapse; worrying about having to navigate too many stairs with bad knees.

Many overweight women report feeling as though entire portions of their day can be consumed with thoughts of food, dieting, and body image, which they know is a waste of their valuable time, causing more emotional conflict.

Vanessa Morris knew the vicious cycle of weight loss all too well, but won the battle with a weight loss of 60 pounds.

Confession #4 on p. 108

Being overweight affects so many areas of a woman's day to day life: her confidence level at home and work; her sex life; her desire to go places, to attend functions with family and friends, the types of activities and social engagements she attends, how she interacts with her kids—even how she shops for clothes. Add to that the social conflict that being overweight is unacceptable in today's society where women are very much judged by their body and beauty. America spotlights on beauty pageant contestants. The skinny, good-looking girls always seem to be captain of the cheerleading team and president of the sorority at college. Even with increased awareness and acceptance of "large sized" models, the majority of advertising and marketing campaigns feature beautiful, stick-thin women that make Marilyn Monroe look fat. Large women's clothes are unstylish and frumpy. Moreover, if you feel like the "overweight duckling" who didn't get invited to the high school prom, it's hard to maintain self-confidence. Whether it is the prom, a bad dating experience, a nasty look, a comment by a stranger, seemingly discriminatory hiring, or failure to get a promotion, such experiences affect how a woman feels about herself and can overflow into all areas of her life–throughout her life! Lack of confidence often leads to a sedentary lifestyle, embarrassment, guilt, more hurt–and–"comfort eating."

Probably the most commonly cited challenge of all is that there is a shortage of time. Today's busy woman has a schedule that doesn't stop. Kids, a career, a husband, family obligations, grocery shopping, cooking, cleaning, washing and paying bills–all consume lots of time. Many women have the additional responsibility of a job. With so many commitments vying for their time, women often put themselves last on the list of people and things to take care of. As a result, many women wake up at 40, take one look at themselves and wonder how and when they let themselves fall apart? Yet most women admit they struggle with the guilt of doing something for themselves when it will take time away from the family. Ironically, the same women who question the cost of joining a weight loss or fitness center think nothing about spending $80 a month for ballet lessons and another $125 for recital outfits!

These physical, psychological, social and time challenges are very real. All of these things make losing weight and keeping it off hard for a woman and she finds herself on the emotional roller coaster that comes along with the ups and downs of the weight loss

Renee Gahagan exemplifies how the social aspects of being overweight can cause one to feel depressed and alone
Confession #5, p. 110

process. The feeling of helplessness one day is followed by a glimmer of hope after meeting someone who has successfully lost weight. The feeling of excitement when starting a new diet that is quickly replaced with a sense of being overwhelmed after just a short period of time. The sense of pride and confidence when weight is lost that is replaced by shame and embarrassment when the weight goes back on again. These polarities pull at the very core of a woman who struggles with her weight.

As one woman who has successfully overcome the struggle said, "I once felt as though I was in a jail but then realized that I was the jailer. I was the one holding the key but I didn't know it. Once I woke up to this reality it was empowering and I simply needed to use those keys to unlock the door and set myself free." It is never too late; you are never too old, never too fat to win the struggle to be thin. This book is going to help you identify the obstacles to successful weight loss and provide you with both the information AND inspiration you need to overcome those obstacles. It will help you unlock your self-inflicted prison and set free the person hiding inside you: the one that has been afraid to come out for years, afraid to dress the way she wants, to express herself the way she wants and should.

So, ladies, settle in to a comfortable chair with a glass of sparkling water and a box of tissues; you're about to get inspired, you're about to learn how to change your life. . . you're about to start your journey to Winning the Struggle to Be Thin.

Do You Struggle to Be Thin?

1. Have you ever kept clothes that once fit you, hoping someday you will get back into them?

2. Have you ever worn a blouse over a blouse or extra-large blouses to hide your excess weight?

3. Have you ever cut the tags off of your clothes so no one could see the actual size?

4. Have you ever bought clothes that are too small with the hope that it will motivate you to reach that size?

5. Do you ever feel as if nothing fits or as if nothing looks good?

6. Have you ever "played sick" for a function or fabricated an excuse just because it was too much effort to find something that would fit or you were just too embarrassed to be with the others?

7. Have you ever tried to hide from someone you haven't seen in a long time before they see you because you don't want them to see how heavy you have become or because you can't remember the weight you were the last time you saw them?

8. Have you avoided eating out with friends or eaten something before going out so others won't see how much you eat?

9. Have you ever told people you were cold just so you could wear more clothing to cover your weight up or said you didn't like the water, so you wouldn't have to wear a bathing suit?

10. Do you ever get a craving for a piece of cake, buy the whole cake, eat some and throw away the rest to get rid of the evidence? Or worse, eat the whole cake?

11. Have you ever postponed a vacation because you believe you will look better in a bathing suit in several months time?

12. Do you resort to food when a personal crisis hits because it is comforting, only to feel guilty after you have overeaten?

13. Have you ever hidden fattening foods or treats from family members so you can eat them when no one is looking?

14. Do you ever think you're overweight because your family has a history of being overweight?"

15. Do you read every "miracle diet" in the hope that it really is?

If you said "Yes" to any of these questions, you are acknowledging behaviors that indicate a struggle within–a struggle to be thin. This awareness is the first step out of denial and your first steps towards change.

Chapter 2

Denial – Hope

Denial: "Refusal to admit the truth or reality."[1]
Hope: "To long for with expectation of attainment."[2]

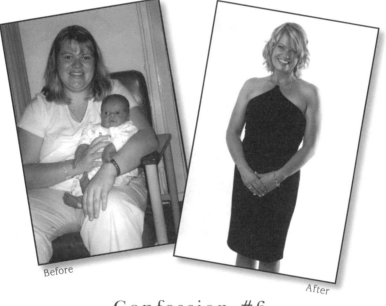

Before

After

Confession #6

Rebel Whale, Tamworth, Australia
77 lbs. lost

I come from a family where my 72-year-old grandmother was still taking laxatives and fluid tablets Sunday night so she could weigh in on Monday at Weight Watchers. She was a life member who lost all her weight and put it all back on. Her entire life she battled to get control of her weight but never won the battle. Unfortunately, 5 years ago she died of a heart attack; no doubt her weight contributed to the condition.

Because of my grandmother's weight problem, I grew up thinking, "Our family just has a weight problem," and that it was my lot in life to end up fat one day.

As a child, anything and everything that happened in my life involved and revolved around food. If I got hurt I got lollies (candies); if we were celebrating we did it with food. My grandfather used to hide lollies in his jackets just for us. Not just one, but four or five bars. And, as my luck would have it, I always had a tendency to put on weight. For example, if I went away on holidays with my grandparents, I could come back kilos (pounds) heavier than when I left.

As a teenager my Mum (who was always very, very slim) would ask me, "What is going on in your life?" When I would respond, "Why do you ask?" she would say, "Because you are standing at the cupboard eating!" Eating was my way of coping, and if I felt stressed, I ate. One time, I can remember standing at my grandmother's fridge aimlessly eating cold apricot chicken and rice with my fingers; I never even tasted what I was eating. I know it sounds disgusting but that is how I was with food.

Prior to having children, I kept this in control through on and off dieting, playing sports and going to the gym. When I became pregnant with my first child, I was 65 kilos (143 lbs.). By the time my third child was 8 months old I was 105 kilos (231 lbs.). I had put on 40 kilos (88 lbs.) over the course of five years while having my children! Although I had always watched what I ate and how much exercise I did, when I fell pregnant I just ate what I wanted when I wanted and did no exercise at all over this time.

What is interesting is that never once in those five years did I weigh myself, nor did I think to myself, "You've gone up a dress size (4 or 5!)." And, because I had access to my grandmothers' wardrobe, I never shopped for clothes. Because I was a woman in her 20's, dressing in 70-year old woman's clothes, my Mum used to say things like, "I wish you would find your style again." (Before I had children, I was a flight attendant and had a great wardrobe.) I may have had a very "trendy" grandmother, but never the less she was 70. Of course, I had no interest in shopping for clothes.

I was in total denial. I really never thought about how much weight I had put on.

The turning point for me was when I went to the park with my children and could not fit in the swing seat. I made a decision then and there that I was going to do something about this. So, the next day I joined the gym. I did it on my own for a while until one day a personal trainer, Mark Frankel, (who is now one of my business partners) came up to me as I was walking on a treadmill reading a magazine and asked me if I had considered personal training. This was the start of my new life. He changed my life that day. I started training three days a week and watched a little more what I was eating. I also started having a fortnightly (every other week) massage.

There were lots of tears and "I can'ts," but I soon started seeing results. Even with those results I found myself ringing Mark and saying I couldn't make it to my training session because my children were sick. Fortunately Mark saw through all that and would say, "No they aren't, I'll see you in 10 minutes," and would hang up the phone. So, teary-eyed, I would get in the car and drive to the gym. And, although I felt fantastic after working out, I literally felt sick before going and some days would use every excuse not to stick with it.

Over the time I trained with Mark, I lost about 20 kilos (44 lbs.) However, the lighter I got, the harder the weight was to lose because my diet still left a lot to be desired. I remember one day whining that I had hit a plateau and Mark said to me, "What did you have for breakfast today?" and I said, "Toast with jam, cereal and a cup of tea." As you can see, I needed some help with what to eat.

Of course, I had tried various diets (probably every single one out there) and would lose weight but I could not keep it off. Once I went off the "diet" I went crazy with my eating again. I was like a shark on an eating frenzy. As a result of this yo-yo dieting, my metabolism was all over the place.

Healthy Inspirations was the answer for me. The food Plan is the only Plan that has worked long term for me. It is not a quick fix; it requires a life style change. It is not a diet, it is a healthy eating plan that you can maintain for life. It has helped me to lose the final 15 kilos (33 lbs.) I really wanted to lose. The exercise circuit is simple to use but gets great results. The massage chair is also huge for me as I was already getting massages.

I am excited to know that this is now my life. I still have tendencies to want to eat when I'm stressed, but have learned and trained myself to go for a walk or do something until the urge passes. I have also learned to live with food; this is an amazing feeling—to know that you can still eat great food and cook great recipes that are good for you.

Now my children have a really healthy attitude toward food and always ask if things are healthy before making choices. In addition, I am now exercising with my kids; I run and the kids ride their bikes alongside. I am so proud to be a fit and healthy Mum and a positive role model to my children.

For me, nothing tastes as good as feeling slim feels.

The Healthy Inspirations Plan has given me back control and that is a great feeling. In fact, it is such a good feeling that I am now the co-owner of two Healthy Inspirations in Australia. It feels great knowing that I am helping other women win the weight loss battle too.

Denial is so hard to admit

Denial is the first obstacle to be overcome if one is to win the struggle to be thin. Consider Rebel's story; she was completely and totally in denial about her considerable weight gain until the day that she tried to get into the swing seat and her rear end didn't fit. Until that very moment though, she said she "didn't notice." Hard to believe that someone couldn't notice that she'd gained 80 pounds but guess what? She's not alone. This book has dozens more stories of women who rationalized their weight problems to the point of complete denial. "I'm big boned to begin with," "I look pretty good for my age," "My husband likes me the way I am," "I don't have any medical problems so I can't be that bad," or "It's my medical problems and medications that are causing my weight gain, not what I eat, drink and the fact that I'm in-active." Family-first rationalizations contribute to denial as well. "At the end of the day I'm too tired to exercise," "I don't have the time; the kids come first" or "If I'm not home for dinner my husband will get angry." These rationalizations provide women with great reasons not to take care of themselves. The reality, though, is that "I'm this weight because . . ." rationalizations are just excuses to avoid taking personal responsibility. The longer one avoids taking personal responsibility for being too fat, the greater their emotional and physical struggles will be—until the "wake up call."

People who have struggled with their weight report going through some period of denial. But, EVERY person who overcomes denial and successfully takes control of their weight reports having a "wake up call." A wake up call refers to an event or happening that moves one out of denial. For Rebel, the wake up call was not fitting into the swing seat. For others it may be a diagnosis of diabetes, high blood pressure, or something much worse. Others will cite the inability to fit into summer clothes, an upcoming event like a wedding, class re-union, or a vacation involving bathing suits, short sleeves and shorts. Still others will share very personal wake up calls like a spouse's vanishing sexual desire, an affair, a divorce or a grandchild saying, "Grammy, you have no more lap for me to sit on!" Whatever the event or experience, it is the thing that sparks wanting to change. Of course, a wake up call for one person may have no effect upon another. The individual must be so emotionally affected by the happening that change becomes a necessity.

> *Tara DeFranco's wake-up call came from her father prior to his passing and helped her to finally begin her weight loss journey.*
>
> *Confession #7, P. 112*

The Power of Hope

Regardless of what caused it, the wake up call provides desire to change and, therefore, the beginning of hope that things can be different. That four letter word, H-O-P-E, is perhaps the single most influential motivator for losing weight. The reason hope is so important to the weight loss process (or any behavioral change for that matter) is that human beings don't like change; change is difficult. However, change is necessary to win the struggle to be thin. Losing weight and keeping it off is all about creating new behaviors: new eating behaviors, new activity behaviors and new social behaviors. Behavioral scientists have nicely broken the change process down into six stages, stages which very much mirror the struggle to be thin process; stages which you must be able to recognize on your journey. These then are the six stages of change.[3]

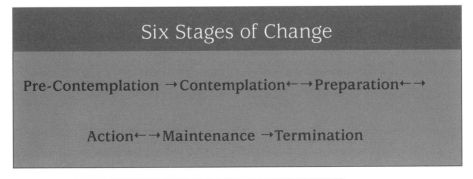

Six Stages of Change

Pre-Contemplation →**Contemplation**←→**Preparation**←→

Action←→**Maintenance** →**Termination**

---

[3] Changing For Good, 1994, Prochaska, Norcross, Diclemente

1. Pre-Contemplation

In this phase, there is no recognition that change is needed. Pre-contemplation is denial. "I don't need to lose weight," "I look pretty good," etc.

2. Contemplation

When moving from pre-contemplation to contemplation the thinking moves to considering change. "Maybe I should consider starting an exercise program" "Maybe I need to lose weight," or "Maybe I could lose weight." This person is no longer in denial, but their language patterns shows a lack of readiness; everything is a "should," "could" or "maybe." There is no real conviction and certainly no plan of action. Everything is in the distant future.

3. Preparation

Entering preparation represents a significant psychological step. This is when one moves from thinking I "should" change to saying, "I will," or "I am going to." For instance, "I am going to start a weight loss program," or "I am going to join a facility." The difference here is the belief of following through with the intention.

In the spectrum of the stages of change, preparation has a very long range. This means that two different people could say, "I am going to lose weight," but one person intends on starting this coming Monday and the other intends on starting at New Years, which is 4 months away. Both are in preparation but are at very different ends of the spectrum.

4. Action

Action means exactly what it says; a new behavior begins. Perhaps one joins a fitness facility, a weight loss program or center, purchases a weight loss book or commits with friends to "start a diet." In our earlier example, Rebel moved very quickly from pre-contemplation through contemplation and preparation and into the action stage—all in one day. This happens for some people depending upon how emotionally stirring their wake up call is.

For others, however, moving from pre-contemplation into action could take months, in some cases years, or may never happen.

5. Maintenance

Immediately upon taking action, one enters the fifth stage of change, which is maintenance. Maintenance is the stage when one has to work consciously at sticking to the new behavior. In this stage, one has to make meticulous plans as to what to eat, strategize about where to go and with whom, and consciously make a commitment to an exercise schedule, possibly even to the point of involving a friend to add a level of accountability. All of these behaviors during the maintenance stage are a normal and necessary part of the change process.

Perhaps what is most interesting is the fact that many people will never leave the maintenance stage; rather they will always have to think about and work hard at eating right and exercising. Individuals who struggle with their weight are actually circling through the stages of change on a regular basis; they fall off the diet or exercise program completely and find themselves back in the contemplation stage ("I should get back on the diet"). Then, they have to move through preparation (I'm going to start on Monday), and take action again, only to find them back at struggling with maintenance. Relapse, although frustrating, is common during the behavioral change process. How many times one relapses before winning the struggle to be thin isn't important but rather, it is how quickly one gets back to the action stage; the quicker the return to action, the greater likelihood of success.

6. Termination

When a new behavior is as natural and routine as brushing ones teeth, one has reached the final stage of change called termination. At this point, reverting back to old behaviors is highly unlikely. People who reach the termination stage are often like the religiously converted; they are so passionate about their revised lifestyle that they try to motivate others to change as well. Another example of reaching termination with the struggle to be thin is the planning of vacations around food and exercise options, ensuring one remains in environments where self-control is possible. When termination is truly reached, an individual simply will not allow themselves to re-gain weight. Many women reading this book, though, whose life has revolved around food and dieting, may never reach termination but are happy to keep their weight under control in the maintenance stage.

After losing 60 pounds, Shelley Branconnier knows that each day will be a challenge because "cheesecake happens."

Confession #8, P. 114

Moving through the Stages

Earlier we mentioned that the "wake up call" startles one out of denial and into hope, but exactly how does change occur and what is it that moves someone from one stage to another? There are only two things that move someone from one stage to another. The first is referred to as a significant emotional experience (S.E.E.), where something recently happened that moved them—in fact scared them is probably more appropriate—into the action stage. Non-scientifically we referred to this earlier as the wake up call.

The second thing that moves a person from one stage to another is education. Perhaps an individual reads an article or pamphlet discussing the risks of being overweight or watches a documentary like "Super Size Me," where a slim, fit vegetarian eats nothing but McDonalds for 30 days, gains a considerably amount of weight while simultaneously increasing medical risk factors. Education is not as big of a motivator as an S.E.E. With daily articles and newscasts on obesity and national television shows like The Biggest Loser, most people know they should be eating better, exercising more and weighing less. With 66% of the US population either overweight or obese[4] it is obvious that most Americans aren't motivated by information. The lack of motivation has to do with the balance of power between the emotions that drive human behavior.

---

[4] "2003-2004 National Health and Nutrition Examination Survey (NHANES)," 30 June 2006, <http://www.cdc.gov/nchs/products/pubs/pubd/hestats/obese03_04/overwght_adult_03.htm>.

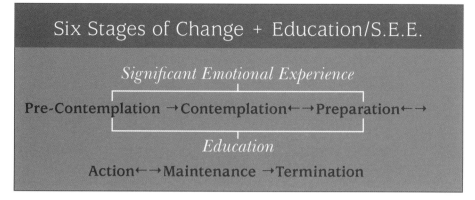

Whether the call to action comes through an S.E.E. or through education, human behavior is driven by emotions—both positive and negative. The S.E.E. or education evokes an emotional response to elicit action. Neuro-Linguistic Programming, which is the study of human communication and behavior, states that everything people do is driven by two emotional forces, the desire to gain pleasure and the need to avoid pain. The need to avoid pain, however, is believed to be a greater emotional force than the desire to gain pleasure. With weight loss, the benefits of looking better and feeling better are always present. However, most people don't begin a

Jennene Kirby lost over 100 pounds after a doctor told her that if she did not lose weight, she would be in a wheelchair before she turned 50 years of age.

Confession #9, P. 117

weight loss program until they experience some level of pain, i.e. bad medical news or prognosis, the potential for feeling embarrassed at an upcoming event, or perhaps finding themselves single again and looking for companionship. This is not to say that people don't start a weight loss program for pleasurable reasons because they do, but more people start to avoid a physical or emotional pain.

Until and unless you find compelling reasons that drive you to want to change your behavior, you won't win your struggle to be thin. You may start a program but most likely will drop out soon after. Identifying specific, compelling reasons as to why you must succeed provides you with an emotional driver, which will help you deal with the inner fears that accompany the weight loss struggle.

Chapter 3

Fear - Courage

Fear: An unpleasant, often strong emotion caused by anticipation or awareness of danger[5]...

Courage: Mental or moral strength to venture, persevere and withstand danger, fear or difficulty.[6]

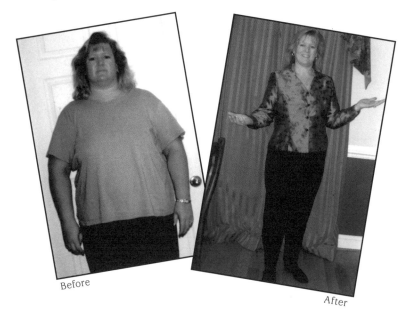

Before

After

Confession #10

Gherri Mort, Winchester, VA
107 lbs. lost

[5, 6] Webster's Dictionary

"Morbid Obesity" was written in my chart by my doctor at my appointment in 2004. Having high blood pressure was another issue that kept haunting me. It was not until I saw those two words together "Morbid Obesity" that made me know I had to do something or I was going to send myself to an early grave. I felt all alone even though I had a tremendously loving family. I just kept beating myself up, saying "How could you let yourself go and get like this?"

In the early 1990's, I had lost weight on a liquid diet, but the weight I lost plus some came right back after I went back to eating solid foods. I had been following different stories on how gastric bypass looked like a way to go for me. But still I hesitated because my insurance would not pay for it. Then I heard news stories of people that were having major problems including death. It was at this point that I knew I had to try to lose weight one more time with a program that used regular store-bought food. I knew deep in my heart that there had to be a program that taught you how to eat right and lose weight.

During the week between Christmas 2004 and New Year's, I was reading the paper and noticed an ad for Healthy Inspirations in Winchester, Virginia. Immediately I checked out the Healthy Inspirations website and became encouraged. Could I actually see the light at the end of the tunnel or was this too good to be true? I called right away and made an appointment for Monday, January 3rd at 1 pm.

As I went through the program orientation, I just knew there had to be some catch. How could eating more frequently throughout the day help me lose weight? Then after Laura finished we went through the cost of the program. I knew that it was going to have a price to pay but I actually sat there and thought "is it worth it?" I could not believe that I still did not feel that I was worth it. Finally, I said to Laura, "I don't know what my problem is, I know that I have to lose weight. I weigh 293 pounds and if there is a guarantee that the weight will come off then I'll sign up."

Healthy Inspirations has changed my life. In just five months after starting the program, I was taken off of my high blood pressure medication. I exercised consistently, followed the eating plan, and met with my consultant three times a week.

Now just over a year later, I am so thrilled to have lost over 107 pounds. Better yet, I have found myself again and also a new perspective on life. I truly feel that the encouragement and guidance of the staff has helped me get to this point. In addition, the friendships with other clients have made a lasting impression on me as well. I realized that I was not alone on my journey. There were more women out there who felt as I did.

Lately I have run into past acquaintances and they don't know who I am right away. I am most eager to let them know that I did it by eating healthy and exercising regularly. I can now see myself continuing on this journey of healthy eating and living. Healthy Inspirations has made it possible for me to take ownership of my life back and pride in myself once again.

> *Shelli Janoff was considering gastric bypass surgery because she was convinced she was going to die. Her final weight loss effort was, however, a success, resulting in 122 pounds lost.*
>
> *Confession #11, P. 119*

Fear—Motivator or Obstacle?

Pain, both physical and emotional, is a powerful motivator for change. Fear is painful, and for both Gherri Mort and Shelli Janoff, the fear of morbid obesity, deteriorating health and high blood pressure provided compelling wake up calls that motivated them to give weight loss one last attempt before resorting to gastric bypass surgery. Many of the women featured in this book note the presence of fear in their wake up call.

Fear, however, often becomes an obstacle for women trying to lose weight. More specifically, the fear of failing again becomes a greater fear than that which provided the wake up call; the fear of telling friends, family or a spouse that you are on another weight loss program. This self-doubt creates a "why even bother if I'm just going to fail" mentality. Two other common fears are the fear of the unknown and the fear of feeling alone in the struggle. Fears often result in one procrastinating change or giving up all together. However, when an individual can get past the fear and generate enough courage the rewards of taking action are waiting.

After getting past her fears, Ann Marie Koohy lost 49.8 pounds.

Confession #12, P. 121

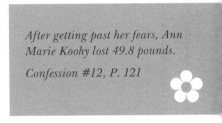

Overcoming ones fears is absolutely necessary to succeed at weight loss, so let's take another example. A woman who has yo-yoed with her weight many times, and is fearful of trying again CAN turn that fear around in her mind to believe, "I may fail again but I want to teach my children to keep trying or I will have failed as a role model; therefore, I must try again." The fear of being a poor role model becomes greater than the fear of failure itself, ultimately providing the courage to try.

For Tara Faro, the pain of not doing things with her family won out over her fears of failure, resulting in a weight loss of 30 pounds.

Confession #13, P. 123

Blame & Responsibility

Having the **courage** to begin the behavioral change process is necessary but courage without taking personal responsibility will result in failure. If you believe you are not in control of your environment, it is too easy to blame external factors for failure. The excuses for the lack of control seem to justify staying fat. For example, buying food for the kids and eating it because it's there. Also, making two meals to accommodate a demanding spouse is too difficult. Perhaps the most common excuse and the one most easily understood is that of the working mother who comes home, cleans the house and shuttles the kids and then feels there isn't any time or energy for exercising. Such mindsets blame other people and events for the inability to do what must be done to lose weight. **To win the struggle to be thin one must shift their mindset** to one of being in complete control of their environment. When the shift in mindset from blame to responsibility is made one realizes things like: A) Junk food and processed non-fresh foods and drinks don't need to be bought for the kids—they get plenty of it at school and with friends; B) Having junk food in the house doesn't mean one has to eat it—it's a choice; C) Gravies, pastas and potatoes don't have to be fattening. If they are, they can be served in side dishes, giving everyone a choice as to whether to indulge or not; D) If one chooses to watch television or visit with friends in the course of a week, time for two short walks every day can easily be made, one before breakfast and one at sundown. Mindsets such as these will lead to success.

Renee St. Clair took control of her environment and her health and reached her weight loss goal.

Confession #14, P. 125

Once you realize you're in control of your environment, the fear of taking action dissipates. The next step towards success, especially for women, is to **put your own health first** because you are the person on whom the others depend. Therefore, if you are not at your best, you probably won't be available emotionally or physically for anyone else. Making this shift is a difficult but necessary step towards winning your struggle to be thin.

Goal Setting

One of the first steps to making the mindset shift in priorities is to establish a goal. A goal is something specific to be attained; it can be something physical (like a new car, a house or a vacation) or it can be a state of being (20 lbs. lighter, 28% body fat, or becoming a size 10). When a woman walks into a Healthy Inspirations and says, "I want to fit into my favorite jeans, she has stated a goal. This is important because a goal represents the pot of gold at the end of the rainbow. A goal won't be reached, however, if it isn't a **S.M.A.R.T. goal**. S.M.A.R.T. outlines the components of successful goals.

"**S**" stands for "**specific**." Wanting to lose weight is too general. Wanting to lose 20 lbs. is much more specific and, therefore, much more attainable.

"**M**" stands for "**measurable**." The scale enables you to determine if you are getting closer to your goal or not.

"**A**" stands for "**attainable**." Is the goal realistic? For instance, if someone has never weighed less than 150 lbs., currently weighs 200 lbs. and decides "I want to weigh 125 lbs., this would unrealistic and, therefore, unattainable under healthy circumstances. Weight loss is challenging enough; setting oneself up for failure by setting unattainable goals is counter productive.

"**R**" stands for "**responsible for self**." If you are not totally responsible for a goal, you may not be able to attain it. For example, saying "I want to do the program so my husband will lose weight," would be setting a goal that you do not have control over; if the husband chooses not to follow the Program there is nothing you can do about it. Setting a weight loss goal just for yourself will avoid disappointment.

"**T**" stands for "**timely**," whether or not the goal can be accomplished in a reasonable amount of time. In this super-busy world, there are many distractions that can easily pull one away from reaching their goal. Therefore, if the ultimate goal will take two years to reach, establishing something that can be accomplished in a shorter period of time will increase the chance for success. You can set a timelier goal, accomplish it and set another one immediately afterwards!

Setting a goal was the key to success for Rose Flitz, who even surpassed her original goal and lost a total of 50 pounds.

Confession #15, p. 127

Getting Clear on the "Why's"

With S.M.A.R.T. goals set, it is necessary to take the goal setting process one step further by clarifying the reasons <u>why</u> it's important to lose weight and keep it off. "Why's" are the driving emotional reason(s) one wants to attain a goal. Therefore, the more "why's" one has behind their weight loss goal, the greater the likelihood of starting and staying motivated. Not uncovering the specific reason/s for wanting to reach a goal makes falling off track easier, and failure is likely.

Clarifying emotional reasons is not a simple process because the human mind is more comfortable with logic than emotion. Women don't walk into a weight loss center and say, "I want to lose weight because I'm lacking confidence with my sexuality" or "I'm totally afraid of failing health and not being around to watch my grandkids grow up." They feel this way, but instead make very logical statements like, "I want to lose weight so I don't have to buy new clothes" or "My doctor told me I needed to lose weight to bring my blood pressure down." Unfortunately, when life gets busy and countless obligations begin vying for time, **logical reasons will NOT compel one towards success; emotional reasons will.** Questions like those below take the very broad goal of wanting to lose weight to the more important emotions behind it:

1. Why do you want to lose weight? *(I want to fit into my size 10 jeans.)*

2. Why do you want to fit into those jeans? *(Because when I fit into those jeans I really looked my best.)*

3. And what exactly is it about the feeling of "looking your best," that you want to re-gain? *(I felt sexier and more confident about myself then. I could wear what I wanted and not be self-conscious about it or have to take a lot of time finding something that doesn't make my butt look big. People took notice of how good I looked.)*

4. And why is getting back to that feeling important to you now? *(I'm not feeling very attractive right now and it is affecting my relationship with my husband.)*

5. How exactly do you think it is affecting your relationship? *(I'm not as spontaneous and my wardrobe isn't as attractive as he would like.)*

6. And what would it mean to you emotionally if you could get back into a more attractive wardrobe and be more spontaneous? *(I'd feel more confident that he was happy with our relationship and me as a partner.)*

Although the woman in this example initially spoke of wanting to lose weight, what she really wants is to feel more confident. By identifying this very emotional and compelling reason to lose weight, she will be more apt to stay focused on the goal.

Often times when a woman falls off track and fails at her weight loss attempt people are quick with judgment, thinking that she was lazy or didn't have enough will power. **Failing at a weight loss attempt, however, rarely has to do with either laziness or willpower.** Rather, the individual didn't have a big enough "why" to succeed. Think about it—if one really believed gaining weight would result in aliens coming and taking their children, a healthy weight would be maintained. The example illustrates clearly the necessity for the "why" needing to be compelling. "Why's" need to be compelling for the long run as well. All too often one has a very compelling, short-term reason to lose the weight, like a wedding, vacation or some other special event. As soon as the reason for success passes, so too does the effort and the weight wins the struggle once again. Long-term weight loss is driven by long-term, compelling reasons "why" success is necessary.

Not only did Christina Escalona want to lose weight, she wanted to feel more confident about her relationship with her husband. Focusing on this goal motivated her to lose 100 pounds.

Confession #16, p. 129

It's Your Turn

The very fact that you are reading this book means you want to win the struggle to be thin. If you are at the point where you have the desire but haven't yet taken action, or if you want to give yourself even greater reasons to succeed, take the time now and complete the exercises below. Doing so will allow you to get clear on your goal, uncover and conquer any fears and provide compelling reasons why you need to win your struggle to be thin.

1. Set a S.M.A.R.T. goal for yourself:
    i.   How much weight do you want to lose (be exact)?
    ii. Do you have a home scale that you can use to weigh yourself regularly?
    iii. Is this weight realistic for you?
    iv. Are you only setting a weigh loss goal for yourself?
    v. Is your goal something that can be attained in a reasonable amount of time?

2. Use the following grid to uncover the emotional and compelling reasons WHY you must reach your weight loss goal. Use the left hand side of the grid to write out all the positive things you will have and experience in your life when you do reach the goal. Use the right hand side of the grid to write out all the negative things you will experience in your life if you fail to reach your goal.

Positives	Negatives

Chapter 4

Intimidated – Knowledgeable

Intimidated: "To be timid or fearful"[7]
Knowledgeable: "Having or exhibiting knowledge or intelligence."[8]

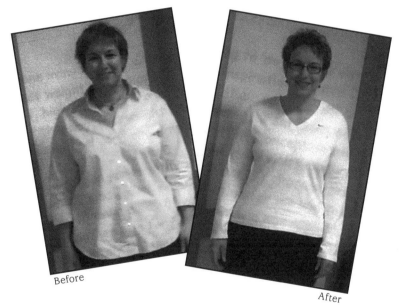

Before

After

Confession #17

Barbara Campbell, Camp Hill, PA
38.2 lbs. Lost

I've done many "diets" ultimately gaining back all that was lost plus more. At 47, I was at my heaviest weight and experiencing joint aches and pains and sleeping in bed was uncomfortable, I had no

---

[7, 8] Webster's Dictionary

energy, high cholesterol and felt unmotivated. I was having an identity battle trying to accept myself this way; overweight with an aging body that was starting to decline, battling against desire to look and feel good about myself, feeling it was unrealistic.

Finding a coupon for Healthy Inspirations, my interest was peaked. I liked what the name implied – Healthy. The ad talked about using grocery store foods, which I liked because I believe that a lifestyle of reasonable eating should be something that is natural and normal. Another plus for me was mentioning the 'stress factor' being a weight issue, which has been in the news lately and quite frankly, I've seen me under stress. Food is definitely one of my coping mechanisms. The ad also talked of encouraging a healthy lifestyle, which I interpreted as lifelong.

But, I was skeptical. I felt I should be able, by myself, to eat correctly and do the right "things"... things that are rather obvious behaviors of a healthy lifestyle and a slim body; things we all know but things I don't do.

Ruminating over the idea of trying to get myself to change my behaviors, I recognized that I really do well with a disciplined, controlled approach with support and guidance. Still holding my coupon, I decided to call Healthy Inspirations. The Healthy Inspirations consultant I spoke to was warm and sincere, however our conversation reminded me of the last plan I had tried. I was very leery of special supplements and diet aids. Tentatively, I set up an appointment to learn more. Fearing my last experience, which had been walking in to inquire about a plan and leaving having spent more than I was comfortable with, I cancelled my appointment.

Still trying to "do it on my own" was futile. After work one day, I was in the neighborhood of the Healthy Inspirations Center I had called. On an impulse, I went in and said I was the person who cancelled her appointment and would they tell me about it now? Well, the women were wonderful and welcoming. I sat down with a consultant who explained the Healthy Inspirations philosophy and Plan to me. She clarified my misconception about diet aids being

*part of the Healthy Inspirations Plan. She outlined the membership
options, daily visits, exercise recommendation and the de-stressing
aid (massage chair, which by the way is out of this world!).*

*Recognizing my hesitance and past bad experiences, the consultant
wrote down the information for me and told me to "sleep on it",
which was very appealing to me. No hard sales tactics or pressure
was applied, another plus. I was presented reasonable, factual information about the benefits of weight loss. The Healthy Inspirations
approach of healthy eating, combined with exercise was exactly what
I was looking for. A sensible, sustainable solution for weight loss
and one that when I reached my goal, didn't mean I had to continue
to purchase all kinds of diet aids to maintain my success. Needless
to say, I signed up the next day! Now, 36 lbs. later, I have energy!
I am wearing smaller sizes. I can skip and run if I want. My aches
and pains have diminished. My cholesterol is down (my good cholesterol is up) and I feel great! My doctor says I should be proud! Can
you tell me what could be better?*

Like Barbara Campbell, **many women don't understand why they
can't do the things they feel they should know how to do when it
comes to losing weight.** Eating healthier foods and getting some
exercise should provide the solution, right? Although that sounds
reasonable enough, a lot of information is needed to understand
the weight-loss process. For some, the technical information can be
intimidating; consequently, many women give up before they start.
This lack of action is the alternative to misunderstanding or misus-
ing the information and therefore feeling foolish.

Another common situation is that many don't understand the science
behind the weight loss equation so they often fall prey to the latest
fad diet. Many of these diets are unhealthy and often lead to doing
more damage to your body than good. A sound knowledge of basic
nutritional concepts and how the body loses weight will enable better
lifestyle choices. Better choices mean gaining control over the
process of weight loss.

Body & Nutrition Basics

Everyday the body expends a certain amount of energy to function, even if one is sedentary. The amount of energy the body needs to function each day is largely based on factors such as age, gender, activity and body composition (what percentage of the body is muscle, fat or water). For example, a larger, more active and more muscled individual will need much more energy each day than a sedentary, overweight individual.

The foods and drinks that we consume provide energy to meet our daily needs. The energy comes from chemicals in foods that are called macronutrients. These macronutrients are proteins, fats, carbohydrates and alcohol.

A calorie is the scientific measurement of energy individuals get from the macronutrients consumed. 3,500 calories equals the amount of energy stored in one pound of fat. Therefore, if you eat 3,500 more calories than you burn, you will gain one pound of body fat. Conversely, if you burn 3,500 more calories than you consume, you will lose one pound of body fat.

All foods and many drinks we consume have calories. However, not all foods and drinks are created equal. In fact, some foods have twice as many calories as others:

One gram of carbohydrate	=	4 calories
One gram of protein	=	4 calories
One gram of alcohol	=	7 calories
One gram of fat	=	9 calories

Food intake is necessary for the body to function. Proper planned food intake prevents consuming excess calories and gaining weight. To maintain proper health, all essential nutrients must be supplied to the body. Learning the basics of nutrition will help you to understand the significance each nutrient plays in weight loss and help you to make more educated choices.

Carbohydrates

Carbohydrates are your body's main source of energy and are obtained in two forms from foods. Starch or complex carbohydrate is the predominant macronutrient in bread, cereals, grains and potatoes. Sugar or simple carbohydrate is found in candy, soft drinks and sweets, as well as naturally in fruit and many dairy foods.

When carbohydrates are broken down by the body, glucose (sugar) is formed which is essential to metabolize fat, fuel the central nervous system, and maintain tissue production. Although all carbohydrate sources eventually end up as glucose in the body, complex carbohydrates are generally regarded as better for you, because they also provide a range of vitamins, minerals and other nutrients, including fiber. Fiber is particularly useful for weight control because it adds bulk, slows digestion and so helps limit calorie consumption.

Simple sugars, which are added to processed foods such as candy bars and soft drinks, are generally rapidly digested and absorbed by the body and can cause blood glucose levels to spike and then rapidly decline leaving a person feeling irritable and nervous. Consuming simple sugars, is therefore, both an all-too-easy way to consume excess calories, and can also result in erratic blood sugar levels, which makes good appetite management more difficult. So, steer clear of high sugar items. The following is a list of the many different names and forms of sugar:

- Brown sugar
- Dextrose
- Fructose
- Corn Syrup
- Honey
- Maple syrup

- Sucrose
- Confectioners' sugar
- Glucose
- Malt, maltose
- High-fructose corn syrup
- Molasses

Proteins

Protein is the body's main source of amino acids and is the major macronutrient in animal foods such as meat, chicken, fish and eggs. Smaller amounts of protein are naturally present in plant foods such as seeds and grains. Amino acids are considered the "building blocks" of the body because they repair tissue, form antibodies to fight bacteria and viruses, carry oxygen throughout the body and participate in muscle activity.

Although there is much debate about the amount of protein the body needs, health authorities generally recommend that protein make up at least 15% of daily caloric intake. For weight loss it can be important to consume a higher amount of protein. Before going any further it is imperative to understand that "higher amounts of quality proteins" should NOT be confused with high-protein, low-carbohydrate diets. These diets encourage too much protein and too little carbohydrate. Because it is impossible to maintain such an extreme eating pattern, these diets ultimately fail and you gain back your unwanted pounds.

For adults to minimize the loss of lean body tissue while losing weight, **you should aim to consume at least 1/2 gram of protein for every pound of body weight.** For someone who weighs 176 lbs., this is a target of 88 grams of protein per day. Proper protein consumption allows the body to maintain as much muscle as possible while burning unwanted fat stores. Maintaining muscles is the best way to help the body to burn more calories at rest (while sedentary). Moreover, protein makes one feel full, and therefore more likely to avoid over-eating.

Protein found in animal products such as eggs, meat, milk, fish and poultry are considered complete because they contain all of the essential amino acids the body needs. Plant proteins, found in vegetables, grains and beans, lack one or more of these essential amino acids and are regarded as incomplete, but plant proteins can be combined in the diet to provide all of the essential amino acids. The challenge with proteins is to consume adequate amounts without eating too much of the unhealthy saturated fat found in many animal protein foods. This is where protein bars, shakes and drinks come into play. Your local health food store has a large selection but it is good to know what to buy and what to avoid. First and foremost find products that provide a generous amount of protein without giving you too much carbohydrate. Aiming for at least 10 grams of protein and limited carbohydrate, say no more than 6 grams of sugar per serving will make for a healthy, filling snack. The snack should also taste good so you will look forward to using it as a snack regularly. Healthy Inspirations has an entire line of bars, shakes and drinks specifically formulated for weight loss, and all products are available for sale to non-members.

Fats

The body needs fat for many functions. **Fats, however, are the highest in calories of the macronutrients and will take a lot more exercise to burn off.** This is why too much fat is detrimental to winning your struggle to be thin. Dietary fats are classified as saturated, monounsaturated and polyunsaturated. Saturated fat, the main dietary cause of high blood cholesterol, is found mostly in foods from animals, and in products made from whole milk (butter, creams, cheeses). Monounsaturated fats are found primarily in plant oils (avocado, peanut, flax, olive, and canola) and seeds. Polyunsaturated fats include safflower, sesame and sunflower seeds, corn, soybeans, etc. When dieting, your daily fat intake should come from monounsaturated and polyunsaturated fats because they are unsaturated and considered better sources of fat for your body. The daily calorie intake during weight loss should consist of only 10%-20% fat.

Vitamins

Your body needs vitamins (A, B, C, D, E & K) and minerals (like calcium, sodium and iron) for the proper functioning of many systems and organs. Vitamins enhance the body's use of carbohydrates, proteins and fats and are critical in the formation of blood cells, hormones, nervous system chemicals known as neurotransmitters and DNA. Minerals are minute amounts of metallic elements that are vital for the healthy growth of teeth and bones. Taking an over the counter multi-vitamin will help the body function at its best during the weight loss process.

Water

The body is made up of 50-70% water. **The water you drink plays two very important roles, particularly during weight loss.** Firstly, water helps suppress appetite naturally by creating a feeling of fullness. Secondly, being properly hydrated prevents the body from sending a false "hunger signal" to the brain. Often the body doesn't recognize the difference between dehydration and starvation, so without proper water consumption, the brain tells the stomach that it needs food. Water also helps the body get rid of waste more efficiently and helps avoid constipation, which is often caused by a change in eating habits—even to healthier foods.

The power of water can be harnessed in two ways: by selecting water-rich foods like fresh fruits and vegetables and by drinking at least 8 glasses of water or caffeine free, sugar free drinks each day. Of course, water consumption alone isn't gong to make one slim but with exercise and the right eating plan, water will help results come easier, healthier and faster.

The Weight Loss Equation

Weight loss is a calories-in, calories-out equation; consume more calories in a day than the body expends and weight gain occurs. Do the reverse and the result is weight loss. Therefore, in order to lose weight, one must burn more calories than has been consumed or consume less calories than one has burned. **The key to successful, long-term weight loss is reducing calories enough to lose weight, but not too much that the body thinks it is being starved.** If you cut calories too much, your body will use lean body mass for energy instead of excess body fat. As was mentioned before, muscle is the tissue primarily responsible for burning calories. People who diet by eating only carrot sticks and salads lose weight initially but end up gaining all their weight back plus some because they have sacrificed muscle and have lowered their metabolism, the rate at which an individual's body burns calories. One pound of muscle burns around 20 calories per day, but a pound of body fat burns just 2 calories per day![9] To keep your metabolism up, the key is to get the body to burn stored body fat, not muscle tissue. Proper fat burning requires a sound nutritional plan with the correct amount of calories.

Proper nutrition means consuming the right amounts of and a wide variety of nutritious foods. Sadly, in today's world of pre-packaged, convenience foods, most individuals are walking around under-nourished. This wouldn't be the case if people ate healthy. In fact, if one could

> *Denise Huffman lost 53 pounds by overcoming her love of high calorie foods.*
>
> *Confession #18, p. 131*

eat all the fresh foods they wanted (fruits, vegetables, meats, dairy and cereals in their natural form) but were not allowed to add or use anything that is manufactured or comes in a package with added calories, weight loss would be far more likely to occur (assuming the individual was overweight to begin with). Combining a low calorie diet with high satiation stops you from eating too much before you consume too many calories. Sometimes, however, the love for non-nourishing foods is a big contributor to weight gain.

To maintain good health and lose weight, begin eating more foods in their natural state, like fresh fruits, vegetables, lean meats, chicken and fish, and natural whole grains, plus low-fat dairy. Further, stay away from bleached flours and refined cereals because they are high in calories without providing the fiber and bulk to help you feel full. Healthy adults should stay within the following servings of each of the following food categories daily:

---

[9] Campbell et al. 1994, Tufts University, Pratley et al. 1994. University of Maryland

- 1-3 servings of meat (including red meat, chicken and fish) and meat alternatives (eggs, protein shakes or bars).

- 3-5 servings of vegetables.

- 2-3 servings of fruit.

- 2-5 servings of breads and cereals.

- 2-3 servings of dairy.

Consuming wholesome, nutritious foods from these food groups each day establishes the foundation for life-long eating habits that will maintain a healthy weight.

The specific number of servings of each food group a person should eat will vary depending upon the total number of daily calories that person should consume in a single day. There are many factors that determine how many calories one burns in a day: daily activity, age, body composition (ratio of muscle to body fat), metabolism and weight all play significant roles.

The average female (assuming good health and no metabolic inconsistencies) burns approximately 11 calories per day, per pound of body weight.[10] Therefore, you can calculate the estimated number of calories needed to maintain your current weight by multiplying your weight by 11. Therefore, a woman weighing 200 lbs. would maintain her weight on 2200 calories (200 x 11). If, however, weight loss is desired, a reduction of caloric intake is necessary. It is generally accepted that a woman can safely lose one pound of weight per week by reducing the number of calories her body uses each day by 500. This is true so long as she doesn't drop below consuming 1,200 calories per day, which is considered unhealthy. Therefore, in the above scenario, this woman would consume 1,700 calories per day to safely lose weight.

There are more accurate ways of learning how many calories one burns in the course of a day. One is called a Resting Metabolic Rate and is done either at a health facility or a medical office. The other is a Basal Metabolic Rate[11] and is done with the use of a body composi-

---

[10] This is an approximation. For an equation that utilizes age, height, and weight, see appendix B.
[11] All Healthy Inspirations Centers provide free Basal Metabolic Rate tests for the public.

tion scale, commonly found at health clubs and weight loss centers. The benefit of using one of these methods is avoiding under or over-estimating caloric intake needs, resulting in faster weight loss.

Whichever method is used to determine daily caloric needs, once calculated the next task is to distribute calories appropriately throughout the day. For 3 meals per day without snacks, take the number of calories that should be consumed each day and divide by three. In the earlier example, 1,700 would be divided by three, equaling 566 calories per meal. If snacks are preferred between your breakfast and lunch, one would reduce their meal calories by the appropriate number of calories in each snack. In this scenario, assuming each snack is 100 calories, subtract 200 from 1700, which would equal 1,500. Next, take the remaining 1,500 calories and divide by the three meals, which would equal 500. 500 is the total number of calories that should be consumed at each meal. By following these equations, calories will be controlled and weight loss will begin.

Knowing the number of calories that can be consumed at each meal allows one to determine portion sizes. Two things are required to determine portion sizes; a calorie counting book,[12] which can be bought at any bookstore, and the ability to read labels.

---

[12] A small calorie counting guide of popular items is located in appendix C at the back of this book.

Reading Food Labels

Food labels can be confusing, often due to the small print and numbers that make them hard to decipher. The good news is that once you know how to read food labels, the information can be used to help lose weight.

At the top of every label are two serving facts. The first is what constitutes a serving size and the second is how many servings are in an entire container or package. It is critical to pay close attention to each of these items to avoid over-consumption. For example, a bag of trail mix may have such a tiny serving size that a small bag provides 6 servings. When one combines the number of servings with the next item on the label, "calories per serving," the numbers are shocking. With 6 servings per bag, a seemingly harmless 120 calories per serving snack ends up being more calories than most dieters should consume in an entire meal – a total of 720 calories!

To simplify label reading, it is best to focus in on just 4 of the listed items; total fat, total carbohydrate, sugar and protein. Anyone with a specific condition that is influenced by other ingredients should be mindful to monitor those label items and take any doctors advice relating to their diet. As it relates to general weight loss and maintenance, monitoring the following items will keep you on track.

Nutrition Facts

Serving Size 2 crackers (14 g)
Servings Per Container About 21

Amount Per Serving

Calories 60   Calories from Fat 15

	% Daily Value*
Total Fat 1.5g	2%
Saturated Fat 0g	0%
Trans Fat 0g	
Cholesterol 0mg	0%
Sodium 70mg	3%
Total Carbohydrate 10g	3%
Dietary Fiber Less than 1g	3%
Sugars 0g	
Protein 2g	

Vitamin A 0%	•	Vitamin C 0%
Calcium 0%	•	Iron 2%

* Percent Daily Values are based on a 2,000 calorie diet. Your daily values may be higher or lower depending on your calorie needs:

		Calories:	2,000	2,500
Total Fat	Less than		65g	80g
Sat Fat	Less than		20g	25g
Cholesterol	Less than		300mg	300mg
Sodium	Less than		2400mg	2400mg
Total Carbohydrate			300g	375g
Dietary Fiber			25g	30g

- Total fat. Any pre-packaged item that gives more than 5 grams of fat per 100g serving is probably too high in fat and should be avoided, when possible. In addition, if a high percentage of the total fats are saturated or trans fat, the item should be avoided, as saturated fat contributes to such dangerous conditions as high cholesterol, stroke and heart attacks.

- <u>Total carbohydrates and sugar.</u> Too much carbohydrate, and, in particular, too much sugar, can raise blood sugar and throw off the fat metabolizing systems of the body and cause energy fluctuations. If total carbohydrate intake is greater than 30 grams per 100g serving, the item will be high in calories. If the total grams of sugar per serving are greater than 20 per 100g serving the item should be avoided.

- <u>Protein.</u> As previously mentioned, you should aim to consume at least ½ a gram of protein per pound of body weight. Meats can easily provide 20 grams of protein in an 80-100 gram serving. An egg will offer about 5 grams from the egg white. Therefore, keeping track of the total grams of protein in each item consumed will be important. The biggest concern with label reading and proteins is with pre-cooked and pre-seasoned items because they can be very high in salt (sodium) and fat. Therefore, even when an item has a high amount of protein, care should still be taken to review the entire label before buying.

Once you know the basics, reading labels isn't that difficult; the challenge is in disciplining yourself to take the time to review labels and then interpret them without going into denial! With a small amount of effort and time, soon you'll be a pro at reading labels, ensuring you stay within caloric limitations each day. With practice you will be surprised at how much food you can eat and still lose weight—a lot of weight!

An 80-pound weight loss was Stacy Pues' reward after learning what it takes to lose weight the healthy way.

Confession #19, p. 133

Exercise, Muscle Loss and Metabolism

The second component to burning excess body fat is regular exercise. Strength training, also called anaerobic exercise, preserves muscles and maintains metabolism for long-term weight loss. After maturity (between ages 30-40), without some kind of strength training, the body naturally loses an average of around ½ a pound of lean muscle mass per year. This age-related muscle loss contributes to a decline in metabolic rate of 2% every decade after age 30. Therefore, just as starvation diets cause a slowing metabolism, so too does aging and it can wreak havoc on weight loss efforts. Muscle loss with aging is why adults tend to gain weight as they age, find it progressively harder to lose weight as they age, and have a more challenging time keeping weight off. Strength training would greatly minimize these three challenges.

Many women may have the misconception that resistance strength training will result in extreme muscularity. This is rarely the case unless someone is genetically pre-disposed to being highly muscular. **Strength training provides tone and firmness to the body while restoring metabolism**, something that is good for the entire family.

Exercise not only helps build and maintain muscle, but it also aids in optimizing bone health in order to prevent osteoporosis. A disease involving low bone mass and deterioration of bone tissue, osteoporosis results in bones which become fragile and are more likely to break. In the United States today, an estimated 10 million individuals have the

Stacey Kubis built lean muscle to burn more calories, consequently losing 23 pounds.

Confession #20, p. 135

disease while almost 34 million have low bone mass and an increased risk for developing osteoporosis. Of the estimated 10 million Americans with osteoporosis, 8 million are women. One in two women over age 50 will have an osteoporosis related fracture in her lifetime.[13]

To optimize bone health and help prevent osteoporosis, women are

---

[13] "National Osteoporosis Foundation: Fast Facts," 15 June 2006
http://www.nof.org/osteoporosis/diseasefacts.htm.

encouraged to take part in weight bearing and resistance training exercises as well as eating a balanced diet rich in calcium and vitamin D. Good bone health will allow one to continue a lifestyle of regular exercise and maintain weight loss long-term.

Today there are a variety of exercise options for strength training. There are traditional machines in a fitness facility; hydraulic machines common at the smaller, women-only centers; body bands, bars and dumbbells that can be purchased at any sports store; even resistance training in the water provides some strength training benefits. It really doesn't matter how one strength trains—just that it is being done at least twice a week. If you are more comfortable seeking professional assistance, visit a local fitness facility or a Healthy Inspirations in your area.

When diagnosed with osteopenia, Deborah Hunter incorporated strength training into her routine and lost 33 pounds.

Confession #21, p. 137

Don't Discard Cardiovascular Activities!

Cardiovascular exercise helps improves health and weight loss by increasing blood flow through the body, carrying more oxygen to the tissues and organs and increasing both energy and stamina. Stamina allows you to do more in the course of a day, helping to burn more calories. Finding a cardiovascular activity that one enjoys helps to maintain a life-long habit for weight control. The chart below shows approximately how many calories are burned per minute with the most popular cardiovascular activities.

Exercise Calorie-Burning Chart

Type of exercise	Approximate calories burned per minute
Aerobic class	11.4
Basketball	9.4
Bicycling@12mph	9.4
Bicycling@15mph	11.8
Bicycling@18mph	14.1
Circuit Weight Training	12.6
Cross-country skiing	9.7
Downhill skiing	7
Golf (carrying clubs)	5.8
Hydraulic Circuit Training	11.6
Indoor Rowing	6.8
In-line skating	10
Jumping rope	9.5
Racquetball	7.6
Running (10 min/mile)	12.2
Running (8 min/mile)	14.9
Swimming (general)	9
Walking (20 min/mile)	4.8
Walking (12 min/mile)	8.2
Water aerobics	4.6

When beginning an exercise program it is important for you to set realistic expectations and begin at a pace that allows for gradual increases in exertion to ensure success. Stepping on a treadmill and running five miles the first day is not realistic. Start slowly by creating some exercise goals that fit in with your lifestyle and level of fitness. In addition, use a heart rate monitor to stay within the proper training heart rate zone.[14] Also, consult a doctor before beginning any exercise program.

Knowledge is power; it allows you to make the best possible, educated and informed decisions–decisions that will affect both your health and your family's health. Knowledge is also the thing that will help overcome any fear of dieting and exercising because once you know what to do and why you are doing it, you feel in control. The next challenge is getting organized to succeed.

> *Shoshana Haas lost 16 pounds by making a commitment to follow a nutrition and fitness plan, learning how to eat and the importance of proper exercise.*
>
> *Confession #22, p. 139*

---

[14] See appendix D to learn more about training heart rate.

Chapter 5

Overwhelmed - Organized

Overwhelmed: "To be upset or overpowered in thought or feeling."[15]
Organized: "To arrange by systematic planning and united effort,"
or "To arrange into a coherent unity or functioning whole."[16]

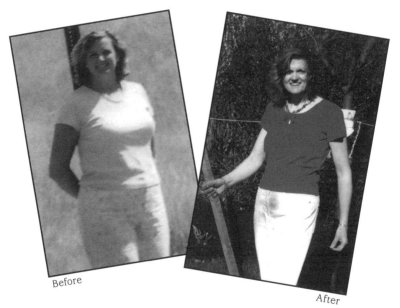

Before

After

Confession #23

Denise Burns, Middletown, RI
36.2 lbs. lost

*I really like myself again. I smile a lot and even sing and dance in
my kitchen with my ten-year-old daughter at times.*

15, 16 Webster's Dictionary

Healthy Inspirations has reminded me to balance what I do for myself and what I do for others. In a nutshell, I learned that guilt is not an option.

Before I joined six months ago, I was in a rut. Like a lot of women who juggle work, kids and housework, there was not much time left for fun. I was down all the time, but when I took the time to do something fun for me the guilt made me feel worse not better. My middle name was overwhelmed.

As the number on the scale crept up to a level I saw only during pregnancy, I knew I had to do something. I made the commitment to myself and joined Healthy Inspirations. In the past six months, I have learned so much more than how to lose 36 pounds. I realize that the best gift you can give to your friends, family and community is to take care of yourself.

I needed to better manage my time so this is what I did. I learned to ask for help with carpools and around the house with chores. I have learned to say thank you even if it is not done perfectly as long as it was done. I discovered the importance of meal planning. For some reason I feared it, like a foreign language and thought it took too long. Now I realize how much time it saves in future trips to the grocery store. I make the time to do the exercise circuit each week, because with the increased self satisfaction and energy I have, I can do more once I get home and I am a nicer person to be around.

One new thing I take the time to do is keep a journal of my thoughts and emotions in conjunction with my monthly cycle. It helps me anticipate the different days I will most likely be tired, cranky or want to throw everything away! As best I can, I plan to rest or have a bubble bath or do housework on those days whereas in the past I may have had a big family party and got stressed and short with others.

My brain is clearer and with my new attitude I can add more to my once full plate. I volunteer to teach computer keyboarding skills to elementary school children after school and became more active in my church. I have more self-confidence and when the journal asks me everyday "What would you attempt if you know you could not fail?" – I have started a list…

I cannot thank the folks at Healthy Inspirations enough for giving my life the kick-start it needed. It has been a true catalyst for change! I know it is up to me now to take the reins of my own life and run with it. I have shared some healthy eating tips with my daughter's Girl Scout troop and with women everywhere and will continue to do so. Thank you for making me feel like an expert on healthy living.

I was on a search back to my old happy self… what I found instead is a new, happier self and look forward to each new day. Thank you.

Organization Conquers Feelings of Overwhelm

Human beings don't like change and, therefore, find the change process overwhelming. This is especially true for adults who are comfortable with their routines and their lifestyles. As a result, it is common for women to de-rail themselves from a new weight loss effort simply because they feel overwhelmed. One common theme in success stories is taking time to organize ones' environment.

Taking time to **clean out junk food** from the home and office is an important first step to organizing and, hence, controlling, ones environments. Removing junk food takes away the temptations that have added to weight gain. For some it is the cookies in the cupboard while for others it is ice cream in the freezer. Identify major eating vices, remove the items and don't bring them into the house while losing weight. If you "can't" throw food out, give it away. Next, having healthy, nutritious foods available and ready for consumption will help prevent reaching for just anything simply to ward off hunger. Personal sabotage occurs when a woman comes home from work and healthy foods are not in the house. Therefore, go grocery shopping often so healthy proteins, starches, vegetables, fruits and dairies are always on hand.

Another aspect of organization is being able to **weigh and measure** calculated serving sizes for each meal. This is going to require three small purchases: a calorie counter guide, which can be purchased at any book store, a food scale for measuring proteins, and a set of measuring cups for measuring fruits and vegetables. You must never "eyeball" foods. Eyeballing causes overestimating or underestimating food portions. Overestimate and too many calories are consumed. Underestimate and the body won't get the amount of protein and calories it needs to stay in a fat burning mode. For those feeling inconvenienced by daily weighing of foods, strategies will be discussed later.

When LeAnn Varano learned to get rid of the junk food and instead reach for healthy choices, she lost an amazing 109.5 pounds.

Confession #24, p. 142

For those incorporating snacks into their meal plan, choosing natural snacks will enable staying within caloric limitations. A calorie-count book can be used to identify possible snacks and portions sizes before purchases are made. Also consider how quickly a snack can be ready for consumption; the faster the better. Again, protein bars, shakes and drinks are wonderful snack choices that are quick and easy and provide a "sweet" snack that many dieters crave.

Meal Planning

Individuals who plan meals in advance are more successful at losing weight than those who don't. A specific written plan is easier to follow and the conscious mind feels more compelled to follow the plan. Therefore, check to see what foods are in the house and then write out the next day's meals, snacks, and times for consumption, ensuring a complete daily plan. When first starting a weight loss program some women plan a week at a time, making a grocery list at the same time. How efficient!

Some dieters need to organize themselves one step further by **pre-preparing foods** to be ready in little or no time. For example, buying a family pack of chicken and cooking it all allows one to open the refrigerator, take out the chicken, weigh it and simply add it to the rest of the meal. This strategy works for either cold dishes or for quick reheating. Proteins are the favored food category to pre-cook, but the same can be done with fruits and vegetables. For instance, clean and cut up an entire head of lettuce or a melon. This is an especially good strategy for singles, as cooking for one every night can be tiring.

Food preparation can be taken another step further by pre-packaging meals. Don't confuse this with pre-packaged meals—i.e. frozen or pre-prepared foods bought at the grocers. You prepare and pre-package the meals so that a meal is immediately available from the refrigerator or freezer. This is a particularly popular strategy for individuals who arrive home late from work. The most efficient way to pre-package meals is by cooking on the weekend when time is more readily available.

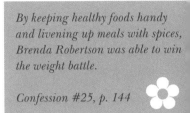

By keeping healthy foods handy and livening up meals with spices, Brenda Robertson was able to win the weight battle.

Confession #25, p. 144

Food preparation and pre-packaging require having the right tools. Airtight containers that can withstand time and a dishwasher are the best way to go. Name brands cost more but typically hold up to freezing and re-heating much better than inexpensive brands. Next, since most of the things being eaten are fresh and perishable, a good insulated lunch cooler and re-usable ice pack is necessary. A mid-size cooler is not too cumbersome but can be used for multiple meals when needed.

All healthy cooking is done by steaming, broiling, baking, roasting, microwaving or grilling, and therefore certain pots, pans and utensils are needed. Select easy to use, easy to clean items:

- Non-stick pans make cleaning up easy.

- A George Foreman Grill™ is ideal for cooking meats while minimizing both the grease and the mess.

- A gas grill (even the smallest table-top size) allows low-fat cooking of meats and even grilled veggies.

- A two-level electric steamer allows you to steam lots of vegetables at once and the clean up is simple.

- A plastic salad spinner makes cleaning lettuce quick and easy.

- A blender for in-between meal protein shakes.

- A food scale, measuring cups and spoons.

- A garlic press is a low-cost item that saves loads of time.

- Pam cooking spray to ensure a fat free cooking surface.

An optional tool is an electric food sealer that vacuum seals foods in bags or special containers. The bags for most machines can be frozen and re-heated in either boiling water or a microwave. This technology allows pre-preparing of foods without the worry of spoilage. In addition, when seasonal berries and vegetables are plentiful and inexpensive, flash freezing and sealing these items provides for year round enjoyment!

Cooking for Variety, Cooking for Life

Organizing the cooking of meals that are flavorful and interesting allows integration of healthy lifestyle choices long-term. Many women start a weight loss program eating only steamed chicken and broccoli. This lack of variety and taste results in succumbing more often to cravings. In addition, women who do not learn how to cook healthfully and tastefully return to their old food preparation and eating habits once the diet is over. Their weight returns as well.

The first step in cooking for life is using the right herbs and spices. Not that long ago only fresh herbs and spices were used in cooking. If fresh wasn't available, there was a dried version of the product.

Today, grocery stores are inundated with sauces, marinades and spice packets for potatoes, vegetables, pastas, proteins—you name it! Like pre-packaged and fast foods, these items are loaded with fat, sodium and sugar. Pre-packaged spices are not needed to make foods taste great. The following is a short list of cooking tips to use until you begin to learn your own healthy strategies from trial and error:

- Fresh herbs are the best. Become familiar with garlic, oregano, cilantro, ginger and dill to begin with. Visit a local organic grocer for a quick education on how to use these items.

- If fresh is unavailable, use Mrs. Dash spice blends, as they contain no sodium and come in 6 different varieties. Explore with other brands so long as sugar and sodium are not in the first 5 ingredients.

- Create meat and seafood marinades with fresh or dried herbs. For ideas, look at the ingredients in your favorite brands and imitate without using sugar and sodium.

- To sweeten a marinade, use sugar alternatives like Splenda™. As an alternative, cut the sugar in half and then add a little baking soda, which neutralizes the acid content, so the sweetness remains the same.

- In lieu of high calorie, high sodium canned sauces and gravies, make your own. For red sauce use fresh tomatoes or canned that have no salt added (Pomi brand is great). Spice with fresh herbs like garlic and oregano. A low-sodium bouillon can be used as a starter; add pureed cooked vegetables to thicken. If cream sauce is desired, add a small amount of light sour cream.

- With egg or tuna salads, instead of using just light mayonnaise, pre-prepare a light mayo-light cottage cheese blend. The texture will blend together nicely with fewer calories and fat in the same tablespoon serving! Another great option for either tuna or chicken salad is to use a small amount of light salad dressing along with some Mrs. Dash (herbal seasoning).

- For "fried" chicken (or anything that is best with a batter coating), roll in low salt bouillon to moisten with flavor, add spices and then roll in crushed, toasted breadcrumbs (or crushed Special K cereal). Bake until crispy and cooked throughout.

- Light mayonnaise, ketchup, mustard, salsa, light soy, fat free half-n-half, light salad dressings, oil, vinegar, and Splenda™ can all be used as condiments. Keep portion sizes to a maximum of 2 tablespoons.

- Finally, extracts such as almond, vanilla, orange, etc. add great flavor and have only a few calories.

May Guenin turned her love for cooking into a love for healthy meals and lost 22.2 pounds.

Confession #26, p. 146

Organize Your Exercise Schedule

Most women today are over-committed and time-crunched, providing the perfect excuse for not exercising. Therefore, it is absolutely essential to organize your exercise schedule. Dieting alone can lead to weight loss but **life-long regular exercise is absolutely necessary for long-term success**. If you think weight loss can be maintained without regular exercise, go back to the discussion of denial in chapter 1.

The key is establishing a set schedule of when to exercise each week. Similar to the kids schedule for karate class or ballet lessons, a regular and realistic routine must be established. Take out your weekly calendar and ask, "If I had to exercise three times a week and treated it like a standing doctor's appointment, what days would I be able to make commitments?" Next, "What time of day can I commit to, morning, afternoon or evening?" It can be different for each day if necessary. Finally, "How much time can I dedicate to my actual exercise routine on each of these days, 30, 45 or 60 minutes?"

Once established, write the entire month's schedule into the calendar. Some women go one step further and place their exercise calendar on the refrigerator door or bathroom mirror then place smiley faces on each of the dates their goal is met. Visually posting goals can be a powerful compliance tool—especially when located where family members or a spouse also sees it on a daily basis.

Changing the foods being purchased, learning new shopping skills, dealing with weighing and measuring foods, exploring with new cooking styles and having to pre-package foods represent significant lifestyle changes. For some, so many changes at once can be overwhelming. The key to controlling being overwhelmed is getting organized and establishing daily patterns; **patterns create consistency**, which is exactly what one needs to overcome the many frustrations that accompany the weight-loss journey.

Kathy Turner found the fountain of youth and lost 24 pounds by organizing her schedule to accommodate her healthy lifestyle goals.

Confession #27, p. 148

Chapter 6

Frustrated - Motivated

Frustrated: "Discouraged in some endeavor; disappointed."[17]

Motivated: "To provide with a motive (something that causes a person to act)"[18]

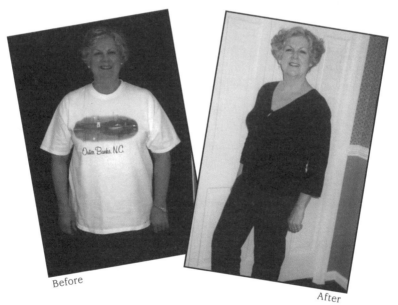

Before

After

Confession #28

Sue Brownlee, Fishersville, VA
30 lbs. lost

I was in my late fifties. I went to the doctor regularly for blood work and my cholesterol was always high, even on medication. I had been prescribed different medications, but always experienced painful side effects. My frustration grew as my cholesterol remained high. My weight was higher than it had ever been and I was looking at my sixtieth birthday on the calendar and feeling old and out of shape.

My mother had been overweight and it alarmed me that I would inherit not only her battle, but her lack of interest in losing the unwanted pounds. I was more than 30 pounds overweight, a weight my body had been used to carrying around for more than ten years.

I had seen an advertisement for Healthy Inspirations in December 2005. When I visited the facility, I was introduced to the most caring staff. They had faith in the program and that I would achieve success with the plan, which inspired me after my consultation.

The fitness center was more than I had imagined. The machines were designed for low impact, which was fantastic since I had not been on a regular exercise program in years. Keeping track of my new eating habits was easy, and almost immediately, I felt a difference in my physical appearance. What pleased me the most was how in control I felt of my newfound habits. The support of the staff on my numerous visits to the facility kept me motivated. My family cheered me on and encouraged me every step of the way.

On February 16th, I turned 60 years old. My family celebrated with me the results that were so evident, thanks to Healthy Inspirations. I had a wonderful day and I felt so good and I had not yet reached my goal! I knew, as I blew out my birthday candles, that I was going to have a wonderful upcoming year.

As I've continued to lose and work out my energy level has increased. I sleep better and have become so happy with myself that I even laugh more. I have been shopping with friends and have moved down several dress sizes since I embraced my new lifestyle. My cholesterol will be tested in May and I'm excited to see the results.

My daughter came to visit after Easter. She looked so healthy, recently losing 18 pounds. She said I had inspired her. I inspired someone to live healthier. What a concept! It made me proud that I had caused a wonderful ripple effect.

I took my daughter to Healthy Inspirations with me on Friday, April 21st, just 15 weeks since I had first joined. The timing was good as I was close to meeting my goal and excited that she could be a part of it. I was overcome with joy when I saw that I had reached my goal weight. After much cheering from the staff, my daughter took a picture of me with the staff, which had walked with me step by step to this milestone.

On the way home, my daughter said, "Mom, when I looked through the lens of the camera, you looked radiant. I've never seen you look more beautiful and it's because you're so happy with yourself." We smiled at one another. Being 60 - no, I'm not old or out of shape. And my daughter thinks I'm beautiful. Yes, it's a good year.

It is easy to appreciate Sue's level of frustration, but **frustrations are pretty much a part of the process**. Almost every woman winning the struggle to be thin uses the word frustrated at some point: repeated failed attempts; not knowing what to do or try next; not being able to lose weight fast enough, or hitting a plateau. Whatever the reason, with weight loss, frustration is never a good thing. The two most common times of frustration are a stalling point (often called a plateau) or a back-slide (where the scale moves in the wrong direction—even when it is a small amount). Whether legitimate, like bloating or water retention during menstrual cycles, or self-inflicted by poor eating or lack of exercise, stalling, or back-sliding is emotionally deflating. Negative emotions lead to negative behaviors and further weight loss obstacles. A woman must quickly get herself re-motivated and back on track if she is to succeed.

Getting Back on Track

Success, not the journey, is what keeps one motivated during weight loss. Seeing the scale move downward is a form of positive reinforcement and is a powerful motivator. Nothing tastes as good as thin feels! So, when frustrated and wanting to say "to heck with the whole process," how does one get back on track? First, be sure to use the organization strategies discussed in Chapter 5. Next, **create accountability**. Accountability means being answerable to someone. That "someone" could be you or another person. Many dieters find using multiple accountability tools to be most effective.

A **food journal** is perhaps the most important accountability tool. People who use a food journal are more likely to lose weight for a number of reasons. Writing down everything eaten and drunk throughout the day prevents excessive caloric intake; makes one think twice before indulging; ensures consumption of the right amounts and types of foods; keeps track of caloric expenditures from exercise; and helps to identify food cravings and situations or events that trigger binge eating. Basically, journaling prevents one from going into denial!

On the following page is a daily journal page sample. (A blank journal page template is available in appendix E.) Each time something is eaten or drunk, record the item and number of calories. Also, keep track of daily exercise in a journal. At the end of the day, follow the directions for sub-totals and totals to determine if more calories were burned than consumed or vice-versa.

Sample Daily Journal Page

Date: Saturday, June 17   **Daily Caloric Limit:** 1400

Food or Beverage Item:	# of Calories:
Breakfast:	
Cereal, high fiber – 1.5 oz.	135
Sliced strawberries – 2 oz.	15
Milk (1% fat) – 4 oz.	60
Coffee, black – 8 oz.	5
Orange juice – 8 oz.	110
Mid-morning snack:	
Banana, medium	80
Lunch:	
Multigrain bread – 2 slices	150
Turkey – 2 oz.	60
American cheese – 1 slice	110
Lettuce – 0.75 oz. (1 leaf)	3
Tomato – 1.5 oz.	10
Light mayo – 0.5 oz. (1 Tbsp)	50
Light/fat free fruit yogurt – 6 oz.	100
Mid-afternoon snack:	
Fat free mini pretzels – 1 oz.	110
Dinner:	
Grilled chicken breast – 4.25 oz.	130
Brown rice – 3.5 oz. (0.5 cup)	110
Boiled carrots – 2.25 oz. (0.5 cup)	35
Spinach salad – 2 oz. (2 cups)	40
Low fat Italian salad dressing – 1 oz. (2 Tbsp)	70
Herbal tea – 8 oz.	5
Water (total daily intake) – 64 oz.	0

Total Daily Caloric Intake: 1388

Today's Exercise: *walked 2 miles at 3 mph*

Approximate Calories Burned: 192

Subtract Calories burned from Daily Caloric Intake:	1196*

*If this total is greater than your daily caloric limit (as recorded above), there is danger of weight gain. If this total is less than your daily caloric limit, weight loss success is within reach!

For individuals who need more accountability than a journal alone, engaging others for
support is a wonderful tool. Identifying individuals who are frequently in your everyday environments (home, work, church, etc.)
provides for the highest level of accountability. Once identified, let those individuals

*When Shelly Rutt realized she was
eating more calories than she was
burning, she changed her ways and
dropped 20 pounds.*

Confession # 29, p. 151

know you are trying to lose weight, and tell them exactly how to best
be supportive. Be as specific as possible with requests. Is tough talk
preferred (I'm going to watch you like a hawk) or sweet talk (I know
you can do this, you're doing great)? Should conversations be kept
confidential or can they be discussed openly? The more specific the
instructions, the more supportive those individuals can be. In situations where family or friend support isn't possible or isn't enough, a
commercial weight loss center provides a tremendous amount of support with knowledge, guidance, a comforting friend during a tough
time or sometimes a much needed kick in the pants. At Healthy
Inspirations support is one of the biggest aspects of the program.

One accountability tool that cannot be manipulated or distorted
is the "S-C-A-L-E;" a five letter word that
many women have a negative association
towards. The scale, however, gets a bad rap;
in reality, **the scale is your friend**. The scale
keeps you on track. Women who participate
in programs where weigh-ins only happen
once a week are more apt to eat poorly im-

*Nicole Evans succeeded with a
strong support system and lost 22
pounds.*

Confession #30, p. 153

mediately following being weighed and then eat salads and carrot
sticks the few days prior to the next weigh-in! This behavior does
not happen when one steps on the scale regularly. Regularly means
every other day, or a minimum of three times each week. If getting
on the scale daily is better for you and won't cause an obsession over
small fluctuations, weighing yourself more often may turn out to be
a motivator.

There are times when the body goes through a phase of decreasing
body fat and inches but the scale remains the same, causing

incredible frustration. This is where understanding body composition (the body's makeup) is important. The body is primarily made of water, muscle, organs and fat. With a certain percentage of each, good health and proper weight are likely. **Having a body composition test done is wise** to discover ones' current state of health and health risks and to provide an additional measuring tool during weight loss.[19]

On her weight loss journey, Tammy Orndorff lost 20 pounds and looks forward to stepping on the scale to see her continuing progress.

Confession #31, p. 156

Body-fat percentage is one of the numbers obtained with a body composition test. A certain amount of fat is vital to daily body functions, as it cushions the joints, protects the organs, helps regulate body temperature, stores vitamins, and helps the body sustain itself when food is scarce. However, as one's body fat percentage increases, so too does the risk for serious chronic diseases such as hypertension, type II diabetes, stroke, breast cancer, osteoarthritis, coronary heart disease, sleep apnea, and other cancers. Below is a grid that tells what **a healthy body fat range** should be according to age.

Healthy Body Fat Range For Females

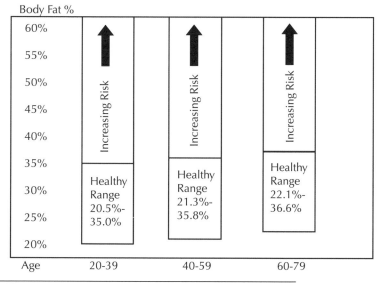

Body Fat %

	20-39	40-59	60-79
Increasing Risk	Increasing Risk	Increasing Risk
Healthy Range 20.5%-35.0%	Healthy Range 21.3%-35.8%	Healthy Range 22.1%-36.6%

Age

---

[19] All Healthy Inspirations Centers offer complimentary body composition testing.

Two other body composition measurements relate to weight loss efforts. The first is **fat free mass (FFM)**. FFM is all the tissue, muscle and fluid in the body that is not fat. Because minimizing the loss of valuable muscle sustains the highest possible metabolism, monitoring fat free mass allows one to protect muscle while losing body fat. The next body composition measurement is **total body water** and refers to hydration levels. Back in Chapter 4 we discussed that being de-hydrated makes weight loss more difficult. If ones hydration level is lower than 50%, more water consumption is needed. Consuming a minimum of eight, 8-oz. glasses of water per day should maintain a healthy hydration level. One additional measuring tool that does not require a special scale is body circumference measurements. This means using a cloth tape measure to determine the girth of ones upper arms, chest, waist, hips and thighs. Having these measurements prior to weight loss allows a comparison during times when the scale doesn't move yet the body is toning and firming and losing inches. All Healthy Inspirations Centers offer complimentary body composition tests.

Getting Re-Motivated

Another way to get through times of frustration is with motivation. For some people, accountability tools are motivating; others feel as if "Big Brother is watching." Many people respond more favorably to the "carrot" approach, staying focused on all the positive things they will attain upon reaching the goal. Every individual will discover unique motivational techniques but there are several very effective strategies that successful women dieters share.

Physically writing out goals and "why's" creates more of a commitment; **re-reading goals and why's on a daily basis** maintains focus and increases the chances for success. In Chapter 3 an exercise was given to identify precise weight loss goals and list out all the reasons "why" success was necessary. This included all the pleasurable things you will realize when your goal is reached as well as all the painful consequences if you don't. If this has not been completed, go back and do it now. To make re-reading a daily habit, tape goals to the bathroom mirror so they can be read while brushing teeth. As an alternative, make a "goals pocket reference" the size of a business card, have it laminated and keep it in a purse or wallet.

Another motivational strategy is to **share goals with a spouse, family member or friend**. Letting others know your goals and their importance accomplishes two things. First, it conveys a level of seriousness for wanting their support. Second, telling others ones' goals adds an additional element of pressure to achieve. Share goals verbally with others or post them on the refrigerator for everyone to see. Make "progress" notes to keep them informed, which will also encourage kudos along the way. A child's report card gets placed on the refrigerator, why not your weight loss report card! The more support one has at work, home and especially at social activities, where food temptations will be at their highest, the greater the likelihood of success.

Another clever and very simple way to stay motivated is to **divide your weight loss goal into smaller, more easily attainable parts**. This is a particularly important strategy when more than 20 lbs. needs to be lost; it makes each step of the way seem more attainable. For instance, if you weigh 181lbs, and the goal is 140, set four 10-lb. goals. Some women like making their goal getting down into the next level of numbers; at 181 lbs. one can think, "just two more pounds and I'll be in the 70's!" These points on the scale prove to be major milestones physically but are emotionally motivating as well. All Healthy Inspirations Centers divide each member's goal into 5 smaller goals: 20%, 40%, 60%, 80% and 100%. Upon reaching each of these milestones the member receives some sort of goodie, like a water bottle, t-shirt, or in some Centers a free facial or cellulite treatment. The strategy is a proven winner.

With the support of her husband's daily messages offering encouragement, Victoria Gillispie lost over 80 pounds.

Confession #32, p. 158

Another way to create incentives is with **non-food rewards**. Women dieters frequently fall into the trap of rewarding themselves with food. "When I get to this weight, I'll treat myself to my favorite restaurant or dessert." Food related incentives are dangerous and will result in self-sabotage. Breaking food associations is the goal, not reinforcing them. Be creative, be kind, and be smart with your reward system. Perhaps the thought of buying a new outfit, getting a pedicure or even a massage will help maintain focus. Such incentives don't have to be material in nature; take a walk on the beach, a bubble bath or perhaps ask someone to take the kids one Saturday morning. Establishing non-food rewards will create both motivation and healthier habits for life.

Consistent use of accountability and motivational tools will help to develop the discipline needed to deal with the stressful situations which are a part of everyday life.

Looking younger and spending more quality time with family was Yvonne Merritt's reward for her weight loss success.

Confession #33. p. 160

Chapter 7

Distressed - Determined

Distressed: "To be in physical or mental strain and stress; being under great strain or difficulties."[20]

Determined: "Having reached a decision; firmly resolved; showing determination."[21]

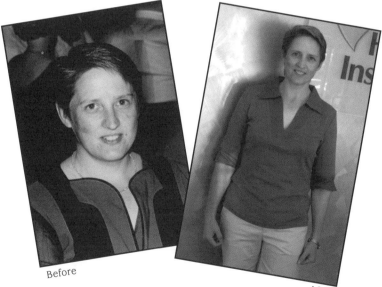

Before

After

Confession #34

Deb Woodard-Knight, Blackwood, Australia
22 lbs. lost

I did not feel comfortable in my clothes, especially at the end of the day and was sick of feeling this way. I felt tired and I reckon I was

[20, 21] Webster's Dictionary

grumpy to boot. I suffered from lots of headaches and wondered whether diet could alter that too.

My main problem was that I had to stop playing hockey, which I had played for 32 years, and I did not know how to eat properly. I was used to eating lots of carbohydrates for competition and found myself getting chubbier once I stopped playing.

I tried a personal trainer for a year and got fit but still did not feel totally comfortable. I was not healthy on the inside.

After chatting with Jodi one morning, I decided to give Healthy Inspirations a go. I liked the way I could eat lots of vegetables (being vegetarian this is easy). I was concerned about cutting out alcohol – I liked a glass of wine with tea, but thought, "If I'm going to do this properly, it's all or nothing".

The rewards of staying on target and on the Plan happened rapidly. I remember being blown away with how quickly my weight went down.

I found it hard when I had lost around 4 kg (8.8 lbs.) and thought it was pretty jolly good, but nobody at work had said anything. I started to feel a bit down. The diet was not easy for me; I had trouble keeping variety in my evening meals and with no feedback from colleagues times were tough. But, Healthy staff to the rescue! Jodi said, "You wait. People will notice after around 5 kg (11 lbs.)." She was right. Another hard time was when I got stuck and could not budge from a weight. Again, the staff here helped by altering my plan slightly and I saw results after a few days!

I am a routine person, so this system suited me. I assign 3 days to attend the circuit and will not budge on those. They are "me" times, which every mother and wife needs. I also treat these times as full on as I can so that I can feel like I am going to get the best results for myself. I like planning my meals. I plan what I have for an indulgence a couple of days in advance and I like to include my family in those times. My family is also eating healthier now.

Reaching my goal was the best feeling. Initially my goal was to lose 6 kg (13.2 lbs.), but I soon decided that another 3 (6.6 lbs.) would be better. I am very proud of myself and my husband is astounded at how I have stuck to the plan without budging – especially since he has witnessed hard times (Christmas!!). My son has also been most supportive, stating one day, "Mum, I reckon your stomach doesn't stick out anywhere near as much now!" Lovely boy.

The inspiration I can offer is: keep positive, keep trying, and talk to people who come in. They all have inspirational things to say and you inspire people too. The staff here are fantastic and have really kept me focused and, well, ...inspired!

Deb Woodard-Knight was experiencing the physical stress of headaches before she lost her weight and found it emotionally stressful when her colleagues were not yet recognizing her successes; more stress when she hit a plateau and again at Christmas time. **Experiencing "times of distress" during the weight loss journey is normal; one must be mentally prepared for such times**. Not being prepared for stressful situations decreases ones' ability to get back on track and increases the risk of quitting. Stress, however, is not an excuse for failure. Unless you win the lottery, don't have to work, move to some remote place, avoid television, Internet and most other human life, stress is simply part of today's world. Stress can be minimized with lifestyle choices, but complete removal is unrealistic.

Stress is not to blame for America's overweight and obesity problem but **stress does influence weight gain**. First, stress boosts blood sugar and insulin levels, which suppresses fat-burning capabilities. Second, when the body is under a lot of stress it lowers serotonin levels. Serotonin is one of the feel-good hormones; with less serotonin, poor mood and even depression occur. Many women then reach for food as a "comfort." A third aspect of stress and weight gain involves the hormone cortisol. Cortisol is produced under chronic stress but is needed by the body to buffer it from stress. When over-stressed the body runs out of the raw materials needed to produce cortisol and then "steals" progesterone to produce the necessary cortisol. That's bad for weight loss because the hormone progesterone is a fat burner and natural diuretic. When a woman's stress level causes a decreased level of progesterone, she becomes "estrogen dominant." Estrogen, which is the opposing hormone to proges- terone, causes the body to hold onto fat and retain fluid. Therefore, when a woman is "estrogen dominant," it causes her to gain and hold onto more fat and retain fluids.

Lisa Leeman conquered her stress and lost 40 pounds. Confession #35, p. 162

People Stress

One of the stressors encountered during weight loss is people. Certainly, it is preferable if the people in your life are supportive and motivational during weight loss, but sometimes the people you love the most sabotage your weight loss efforts. You may think you don't have to worry about that, that none of your friends or family members would want to sabotage your efforts. That may be true, but before dismissing the thought, let's explain.

A saboteur is a person who actively undermines your weight loss efforts. Sadly, sabotaging happens most often when someone close to you feels threatened by your new lifestyle or about what it may mean to the relationship between you both if you become more slim and fit. The saboteur may complain about the new food choices in the house, yell about time away for classes or exercise or even say you're bound to fail. Some less overt sabotaging behaviors include the person recalling past weight loss failures, buying junk food for the house, eating high caloric foods in front of you, "innocently" offering junk foods, or perhaps suggesting that it's okay to cheat. For instance, "You look great, come on, one won't hurt you," or "Let's celebrate, I haven't seen you in so long."

Although a **saboteur** is often oblivious to their negativity, sabotaging behaviors–both conscious and unconscious–hinder success. The best course of action with a saboteur is to sit down with the person in a quiet, non-intimidating environment and have a heart-to-heart talk. Sometimes it will be difficult for close friends and family members to admit they have been negative because it forces self-reflection as to why they don't want you to succeed. In some instances, a third party must be brought in to "referee" the conversation. In the end, you may have to deal with the reality that a saboteur remains "in your camp," and alternative strategies must be found. Regardless of the types of surrounding influence, ultimately you are responsible for success.

Another stressful personality is **the enabler**. An enabler doesn't overtly try to create failure but rather knowingly stands by, supports, or encourages bad weight loss behaviors. This is often done because good friends, family or spouses don't want to see you suffer.

For example, suppose a married couple goes out to dinner. The wife has been doing great on her weight loss program, having lost 20 pounds and is half way to her goal. While looking at the menu she says, "I think I'll get the fried clams tonight," which just happen to come with

Though friends and family sometimes discouraged her decision to lose weight, Shirley Jones did not give up on her goal to slim down

Confession #36, p. 164

french-fries. Both know this is not a healthy selection. In fact, the reason she mentions the selection aloud is to see what the husband's reaction would be. The enabler would either say nothing–which is silently giving that person permission–or he may actually say, "go ahead, you deserve it." Either the silence or the enabling comment is not what is needed for weight loss success. Rather, the husband should say, "you know honey; you're over half way to your goal and looking so great. If you eat that, tomorrow you are going to get on the scale and regret it. Why don't you celebrate by making a healthier selection and instead, treat yourself to a manicure tomorrow." This type of comment keeps the dieter on track. Another example might be during a vacation. The wife says, "I don't know how to use the fitness center at the hotel, I think we'll get plenty of exercise sight seeing." An enabler might say nothing or actually agree. Again, this is not what is needed. Rather, encouragement to exercise helps to deal with the stress of unfamiliarity. "Let's go figure it out together," or "Let's go for a 30 minute power walk now, that way we'll feel great knowing we've gotten our exercise in for the day."

Empowering and supportive comments do not come naturally to an enabler. Communicating to them that support is wanted is the first step. Second, explain to them what an "enabler's" behavior involves. Third, coach them in the type of comments and support that is preferred. Finally, recognize that there will still be times when old behaviors return and a new solution will have to be worked out.

Another "people stressor" is children. Typically, children in the household create two challenges. One is having junk food in the cupboards for lunches and snacks. Two is arriving home late from work and having to take the kids to McDonald's, order out for pizza or some other fast food option.

A weight loss program gift certificate from her daughter gave Mildred Gehrke her start to losing 30 pounds.

Confession #37, p. 166

Both of these situations require mom to watch the kids indulge without doing so herself, which is stressful. First, realize that junk food does NOT have to be purchased for children; they get enough of these foods at school, friends' houses and social functions. Kids won't like the absence of their favorite fattening and sugary substances, but the Department of Children, Youths & Families is not going to come take children away for "no junk food abuse." Much to the contrary, kids are healthier with eating fruits, vegetables and nuts as snacking options. Second, if junk food is purchased or kids are taken out for fast food, strategies that will fit one's level of discipline must be created. For instance, designate a special cupboard in the kitchen for all these items, avoiding a face-to-face encounter with the package of Oreo cookies while preparing dinner. Get carry-out for the kids instead of eating at the fast food restaurant, making it much easier to be home preparing a healthy meal instead of being tempted by the kids' french-fries while watching. Finally, know

As Nancy Eagle worked to lose 41.4 pounds, the support from her kids helped her stay focused.

Confession #38, p. 168

that kids aren't always a roadblock to weight loss efforts. In fact, some kids support and encourage their moms because they want them to be healthier and live longer.

Environmental Stress

A second type of stress that is encountered is environmental, and this does not refer to the world's pollution levels. Personal environments are those real-world situations such as parties and social functions, restaurant and fast food dining, and vacations, all of which are perfect breeding grounds for stress during weight loss. For one thing, such situations alter one's routine; routine is what people need when trying to lose weight. Second, in any type of social environment the peer pressure to enjoy oneself is present at both the spoken and unspoken level. Some of these environments will prove to be most challenging and will require success strategies.

Socializing is synonymous with eating; whether it's an office party, a wedding, a graduation or even a funeral, food is the primary event that brings people together. When people are eating in a social setting they expect and encourage other's to eat with them. There are ways, though, in which social activities can be enjoyed while staying on track.

Before the Party

- When attending a party at the home of friends, contact them ahead of time and let them know you have certain dietary restrictions. With chronic conditions like high blood pressure, cholesterol and diabetes, it is not unusual for people to have special dietary requests.

- If comfortable with the host, specifically ask to have certain healthy foods available.

- Let others at the party know your goal is to "stay on track" and ask them for help and support. Most people will be cooperative, respectful, and encouraging.

- When attending a cocktail party, eat a meal before going, reducing temptation for hors d'oeuvres.

Food Selections

- For a potluck event, bring a healthy main course, like a chicken and lettuce salad with a separate container for dressing.

- Try to consume the leanest protein source available as well as lots of fresh vegetables.

- Simply say, "No thank you," to foods rich in fat or sugar.

- Try to avoid any potatoes, starchy vegetables and breads.

- If certain foods are only available with sauces and gravies, try to remove as much of those toppings as possible and/or decrease the portion size to account for the extra fat and calories.

- If unhealthy foods can't be resisted, eat all the healthier selections on the plate first so you fill up. If "needed," take a bite or two of the unhealthy choices. Often taste buds are satiated after one or two bites.

- Eat slowly and leave any unwanted food. "Cleaning" your plate is not necessary to show that a meal has been enjoyed.

Dessert Selections

- When bringing a dessert, be sure to make a nice bowl of fresh fruit that is low in calories and fat. Always choose the fresh fruit over any other option.

- If no fruit is available and dessert is a "must," select the least fattening, least caloric item. Further, take the smallest possible piece and take only one or two bites.

After the Party

- If time permits, go out for a walk.

- Regardless of how convincing the host or hostess is (especially your mother or in-laws), either do not take food home unless it is healthful or take it home but give it away or simply throw it out. Know your own level of discipline!

- If you do over-indulge, get additional exercise the next day, be extra good about your food selections for the next two days, and consume extra water.

- Learn from experience and use better strategies for the next social engagement.

Restaurant dining can also be challenging. Many people feel awkward making special requests regarding meal preparation. Also, regardless of what is requested, there is little control over how a chef ultimately prepares a meal. Still, because eating out is such a big part of today's culture, both pro-active and re-active strategies must be developed.

Before Ordering

- When possible, try to select a restaurant that offers healthy choices.

- If possible, turn away the waiter bringing a basket of bread. If not, keep the bread away from where you are sitting.

- Be ready to avoid temptation and able to say no to things like grated cheese or a side dish of pasta.

- Start with an 8-ounce glass of water to fill you up while reading the menu.

- Try to focus on enjoying the company, not on the food and beverages.

Appetizers

- For an appetizer, find a broth-based soup, shrimp cocktail, or clams on the half shell; ask for extra lemon and use a minimal amount of cocktail sauce.

- Stay away from stuffed mushrooms, stuffed clams, etc, as these foods have lots of breading and fat.

- When ordering a salad, ask for no croutons; order the salad dressing, preferably oil and vinegar or light dressing, on the side

- If you overindulged in the appetizers, when the entrée comes, immediately half the portion and ask for a doggie bag. Get the food off your plate!

Main Course

- Be confident and aggressive when ordering. Don't be embarrassed to make special dietary requests, as many people do this for medical reasons.

- Stay away from sauces; barbeque, Alfredo, and even red sauce can be loaded with fat and sodium. If you must have pasta, choose a marinara sauce.

- If the meal comes with some kind of sauce on it, send it back or scrape if off before eating.

- Choose grilled meats, chicken, fish, and vegetables.

- Don't be afraid to request that vegetables be prepared without any butter or seasoning.

- Stay away from the pastas if possible. If pasta is only side dish available, half the serving.

- If a pat of butter comes on the baked potato, take it out, and squeeze lemon on the potato instead; it's delicious.

Another aspect of eating out is dealing with **fast food**. Fast food chains are certainly adding healthier selections to their menu, but high sodium, high fat and high caloric choices are still the norm. Even selections that boast "low fat" are not necessarily

Learning how to incorporate a weight loss plan into a hectic, "on the-run" lifestyle enabled Susan Thomas to lose 23.8 pounds

Confession #39, p. 170

healthful. Special requests are more difficult at fast food places and, therefore, consumption should be minimized, especially during weight loss. However, there are some simple strategies to minimize fat and calories.

Leigh Bruffy lost 28 pounds by learning how to eat at social situations and still maintain her weight.

Confession #40, p. 172

- Look for items that are grilled, not fried.

- Always order a plain sandwich or burger. This allows for control of condiments and usually results in a fresher sandwich made to order.

- If the selection comes with cheese, ask for it to be removed all together. Cheese is high in calories and fat and is best to avoid during weight loss.

- Immediately remove half of the sandwiches bread. Either fold the entire sandwich in half so bread is on either side or eat it like it like a piece of pizza.

- Only order fast food soups if they are low sodium.

- Be mentally prepared to say "No," to up-sell questions like, "Would you like fries with that," or "Would you like to super size that meal?"

- Avoiding french-fries altogether is best. If unavoidable, split a small order with someone.

Vacations are a wonderful part of our lives. Unfortunately, vacations throw us out of our day-to-day schedules and routines for a number of days or weeks. Learning how to successfully go on vacation without coming home having gained 10 pounds is a must! The general rule for surviving vacations is proper planning.

Plan the right type of vacation

- Know what food selections and exercise options are available prior to making your trip arrangements.

  ▲ For instance, cruises are notorious for packing on the pounds but many cruise lines today offer trips that have a focus on activities both on board and with daily excursions. In addition, most ships now have a "spa" or "healthy" selection for all courses of meals.

  > *Pamela Mott has lost 20 pounds thus far and is learning how to get back on track after an event or vacation throws her off course.*
  >
  > *Confession # 41, p. 174*

  ▲ The same is true for destination vacations. The bottom line is that vacations offering a higher level of activity and healthy food options are available!

Pre-plan options

- When not in control over the destination, do some research before arriving and pre-plan both food and exercise options.

  ▲ Find out if the hotel has a fitness center or offers aqua aerobics classes in the pool.

  ▲ If neither of those is available, ask about a local fitness center. Many club organizations have reciprocal club usage programs or reduced day-rate fees.

  ▲ Inquire about walking paths.

- When planning activities and sightseeing, select things that are physical or have a lot of passive exercise involved. Even walking through a museum for 4 hours is better than sitting on a bus tour.

- One way to ensure getting enough activity is to wear a pedometer and get in 10,000 steps per day.

- When it comes to meals, call ahead to the hotel restaurant and ask to have a menu e-mailed or faxed. Go over it ahead of time to find healthier options as well as identifying items that should be avoided. When temptations can be identified ahead of time, it will be easier to create a success plan.

- Ask the front desk to recommend local restaurants that are known for healthier selections and begin formulating your itinerary around those places.

Pre-plan travel time

- Ensure that enough "road foods" are packed until the travel destination is reached. Airport and rest area foods are loaded with fat and calories and most have no nutritional value.

- Cut up fresh veggies, pack fruits that will travel well, bring a sandwich that has a healthy protein source or simply pack several hard-boiled eggs.

- Bring a soft-sided cooler with a re-freezable ice pack, which can be re-stocked for the trip home.

- Bring plenty of water, avoiding paying $2.50 for a 12-oz bottle in the airport.

- Bring plenty of protein bars to get through both the travel time and the vacation.

- While waiting for trains or planes, instead of sitting, get up and move! Wear comfortable shoes or sneakers and loose fitting clothes. Walk up and down the airport or pace on the train platform.

- When on long road trips, take 20 minutes and power walk around the parking lot at rest areas. You may look foolish, but you will feel a heck of a lot better at the end of the day.

Pre-plan alcohol and food cheats

- When going away on a 7-day vacation (or longer), determine ahead of time how many alcoholic drinks will be allowed and how many desserts (if these are your "vices").

- Next, allocate those "cheats" out over the course of the vacation.

- Write those "self-policing rules" down and share them with travel companions, asking them for support, if necessary.

Have a fall-out plan

- The worst thing to do while on vacation is fall into, "the heck with it" attitude. This is when your mind rationalizes that since there has been two bad days all caution can be thrown to the wind for the rest of the vacation; worry about getting back on track next Monday! This NEVER works; vacationers that gain too much weight get depressed and Monday never comes.

- Enlist travel partners to be your "eyes" and give them permission to pull you back on track if necessary.

The Importance of Stress Reduction

One also needs to learn how to reduce stress levels. The word stress implies force or tension. When it comes to the body, some people feel stress in their neck and shoulders, some get headaches, others feel a pit or indigestion in their stomach. All of these symptoms are because stress builds up in the body and is now manifesting itself physically. When left un-treated, "strugglers" reach for food as a "comfort" through difficult times. This is why stress reduction is important. There are dozens of books, audios and videos on the topic of stress reduction and investing in some of these materials will provide many tools and strategies. In the meantime, to assist your weight loss efforts, there are stress reduction basics of which you should know.

Exercise is one of the best forms of stress reduction available. Increased physical activity burns off cortisol levels in the body and will reduce tension both chemically and physically. Think about it, when the kids are bouncing off the walls, they're sent outside to run around and "burn off" some of their energy. Stress is nothing more than pent up energy in an adult body—it just happens to be a negative energy. Whether it is positive stress (an important upcoming event) or negative stress (problems at work), participating in physical activity will reduce stress levels and do the body good at the same time, giving exercise a dual purpose.

There are times when one simply doesn't have the physical or emotional energy to move! During these times, another great stress reduction option is to **pamper oneself** with a little indulgence. Getting a massage, a new hairstyle, a facial, a manicure or a pedicure are all things that can de-stress and make one feel and/or look better. Of course, spending money to pamper oneself isn't necessary. Turn on some relaxing music, lock the bathroom door, and take a nice, hot bubble bath. All of these things are kind on the body and calming to the mind. Another way to de-stress is to have some quiet time. This may mean sitting on the back porch watching birds at the feeder, taking the dog for a walk in the park or on the beach, finding a comfortable chair to curl up in and reading a good book or participating in some deep breathing and meditation exercises. There are endless possibilities to getting in some quiet time; the most important thing is that they are enjoyable.

Having made the choice to lose weight, you will encounter both people and environments that prove to be stressful during the struggle to be thin. **Winning the struggle requires you to display determination in using the strategies for life, not just when dieting**.

Chapter 8

Embarrassed - Humbled

Embarrassed: "To experience a state of self-conscious distress; to be in doubt, or perplexed."[22]

Humbled: "Not arrogant; reflecting, expressing or offered in a spirit of deference."[23]

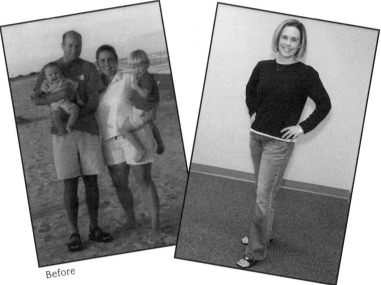

Before

After

Confession #42

Amy Horst, Lancaster, PA
31 lbs. lost

[22, 23] Webster's Dictionary

Last summer, I received an invitation to my 15-year high school reunion. My childhood friends decided to go, but I made up an excuse and said I wouldn't be joining them. If I had been honest with them and myself, I would have admitted that it was because I was embarrassed about my appearance. I was 32 years old and 40 pounds overweight.

I have struggled with my weight for as long as I can remember. I've had many ups and downs over the years and my weight often fluctuated with my emotional highs and lows. Last summer was a low for me, probably lower than even I wanted to admit. After stepping back, looking at my wonderful husband and my two amazing children I realized that I wanted to be there for them, emotionally and physically. I wanted to run in the backyard with my kids and not become winded, I wanted to swim in the pool and focus on my kids, and not how insecure I felt in a bathing suit. I wanted to feel good about the woman, mother and wife that I am. Being forty pounds overweight was not healthy for me, emotionally or physically. I knew it was time for a change.

I have tried various weight loss programs in the past. I always lost weight but never reached my goal. I would become frustrated and give up. Inevitably, the pounds would creep back on. I wanted a permanent change. After calling around to various places, I decided to give Healthy Inspirations a try.

I liked Healthy Inspirations immediately. They taught me how to meal-plan with healthy choices; and checking in three times each week keeps me motivated and on track. The exercise circuit never feels intimidating or overwhelming. Most importantly, the support and encouragement of the staff has been an essential part of my success.

For me, the best part of Healthy Inspirations is the camaraderie. As with any weight loss program there are ups and downs, and when I go to the center to check in, it isn't always a "good" day. But I always know that the staff and other women in the program will support me. While we are all at various stages in the program, we are all there for the same reason. We have walked in each other's shoes and while exercising, we often talk about our highs and lows and offer support to each other. There is always someone to make a suggestion or encourage me, I never feel alone.

Four months later and thirty-one pounds lighter (9 more to my goal!) I feel like a new woman. I have more energy, more stamina and a lot more smiles for my family. Not only do I feel physically rejuvenated, I also feel emotionally healthy.

Issues with food and weight have long been a challenge for me. It hasn't been easy and I have searched high and low for a solution. Because of Healthy Inspirations, weight loss has not been a diet but rather a journey of self-discovery. I have learned a lot in the past four months not only about food and exercise but also about myself.

I initially decided to make a change because of my family; I wanted to be healthy for them. Healthy Inspirations taught me not only how to eat and exercise properly, but also how to be accountable to myself for a lot of decisions in my life. I learned that I want to be healthy for me.

Kathleen Wilson overcame the embarrassment of gaining back pounds lost from a previous attempt and has now lost 65 pounds.

Confession #43, p. 176

No One Likes Embarrassment

For Amy Horst, Kathleen Wilson, and many women, embarrassment drove them to take charge of their lives and lose weight. In this respect, embarrassment was a positive thing. Unfortunately, embarrassment can be a major obstacle to weight loss success, occurring most often after a woman succeeds at losing some or all of her weight but subsequently falls off track, resulting in the scale's creeping upward. First there is the embarrassment of not being able to maintain control of one's eating, which often leads to self-pity and more eating; next is the embarrassment of asking for help, so none is sought;

this is followed by the embarrassment of getting back on the scale, so it is avoided; finally there is the embarrassment of the regained weight. These embarrassments often cause women to do two things. First, play mind games with themselves; second, return to denial.

Take the situation where a woman has friends whom she doesn't often see. At the last meeting, the woman had lost 40 lbs. but has since gained half of it back. She's embarrassed and upon learning that she will soon see them, she agonizes over what to wear that might hide the weight re-gain. She thinks about what passing comment could be made that would provide some "excuse" for the backslide or perhaps even fabricates a reason NOT to see them. These types of mind games don't fool anyone—not even the struggler.

The second scenario is worse. The feelings of embarrassment are so overwhelming that the woman goes into a mode of denial. "I still look good, at least much better than before," "I deserve a little break after working so hard; I can't deny myself the things I love forever," or "I'll get back on track Monday." Monday comes and goes and the elastic waistband pants find their way back into the drawer; next, shirts aren't being tucked in. Of course, the scale collects dust in the bathroom closet. In both these scenarios, the woman has fallen out of maintenance and into a relapse. Remember, relapse is a normal part of any behavioral change. Unfortunately, knowing relapse is "normal" does not remove the embarrassment or guilt associated with regaining weight.

What Causes Relapse?

Women who yo-yo with weight identify four major mindsets that contribute to relapse. The first is **"justified cheating."** With this mindset the woman finds herself saying things like, "I'm over half way to my goal, I deserve a piece of cake," or "I've worked so hard I deserve a night off." The problem, however, isn't taking one night off; if "cheats" were infrequent, gaining weight wouldn't reoccur. The problem is the foods one cheats on reignite desires for unhealthy foods. The individual focuses on how good the food tastes and justifies cheating again the next day–and the next day . . . One night of justified overindulgence becomes a week and then a month and before long all the lost weight has been re-gained.

Next is the **"all or nothing" mindset**. This mindset frequently sets in after a period of justified cheats, particularly during vacations. With this mindset, the individual is either on the diet or not; there is no middle ground. Therefore, after a Thursday evening of poor eating the individual thinks, "Well, I'm off the diet now; I may as well just re-start on Monday." For some this mindset becomes a daily struggle where eating an unhealthy breakfast results in an "I've blown it now, I'll try again tomorrow" attitude. In all of the preceding, the individual has forgotten that eating healthily is a lifestyle, and every meal and every day counts. It is not an all or nothing process but rather a balanced approach.

The **"why bother" mindset** presents itself when weight has been regained or when a plateau is in effect. In this mindset, the attitude is, "this is just too much work, so why bother." Other frequent comments are: "I should eat and enjoy life; you never know, I could get killed by a car tomorrow so why not have what I want?" "What can I say, I'm fat, and I've always been fat, why try and fight it. My pants are tight, but I'm emotionally comfortable." "My friends are fat, my husband doesn't care, and, what the heck, I still have fat clothes." Many women express this attitude publicly, but privately continue to struggle with thoughts of wanting to be thin.

Fourth is the **"It's only . . ." mindset.** For instance, "it's only 10 pounds; I can lose that again when I want" or "I've only gained a few pounds and I still look good." This mindset is most often present immediately after individuals reach their weight loss goal. While feeling good about themselves, the way they look, and their recent accomplishment, a false level of confidence is created. This often leads to more justified cheating and for many the downward spiral begins again.

All these mindsets are roads to failure. Failure leads to guilt, depression, and more eating and weight gain—again. Identifying these mindsets is one thing but the underlying question women who struggle with their weight can't seem to answer still exists: "Why can't I keep the weight off?" It's a valid question. One would think that after losing weight and feeling so good physically and emotionally that an individual would never relapse and regain the weight again. Such an accomplishment is easier said than done; many women continuously sabotage their weight loss efforts.

Webster's Dictionary defines sabotage as "An act or process tending to hurt someone or something." Two things are of particular interest with that definition. One, sabotage can involve either a single act or a process, which is a series of pre-contemplated events with a specific goal

After putting off a weight loss plan and struggling at the start, Lesley Reilly succeeded in losing 31.5 pounds.
Confession # 44, p. 178

in mind. Second, sabotage results in some form of hurt. This means that regardless of how much an individual may say, "I didn't mean to sabotage my efforts," or "I don't know why I ate the entire bag of chips," self-sabotaging one's weight loss efforts is actually a thought process executed by an individual with the intention of hurting themselves, albeit unconsciously.

Eating Associations

The stimulus-response aspect of human behavior provides insight into self-sabotage. For every behavior you exhibit, there is a response from the people around you; when a good response is generated, a positive association to that behavior is created; when a bad response is generated, a negative association to that behavior is created. **All behaviors, therefore, are created no differently than Pavlov's theory**: Make dogs hungry and then feed them while ringing a bell. Do this over and over again and pretty soon when the bell is rung the dogs salivate. The result is the creation of an association for the dog that "the ringing bell means I'm going to get fed."

Every time one sabotages weight loss efforts (typically by eating junk foods or too much food) it is done because a situation triggered something emotional and the individual turned to food for comfort. Analogous to Pavlov and his dogs, the individual gets stressed and grabs for cookies, gets frustrated and eats an entire container of ice cream, or gets depressed, says, "to heck with it," and eats an entire bag of chips. This results in eating associations.

Eating associations are created at a very early age and the memory of when the association was created and the trigger that causes the behavior is unconscious. For instance, a mother gave her toddler a cookie every time something traumatic occurred; as an adult this individual reaches for cookies every time there is stress. Unfortunately, because eating associations happen at such an early age, one cannot logically figure out why they sabotage their efforts nor can they seem to stop themselves before or during the sabotaging behavior—even when their conscious brain is telling them not to do it. The good news is that you can stop sabotaging your weight loss efforts by identifying your eating associations and then design a plan to stop the cycle.

There are **three key factors influencing eating associations** of which one must become aware. 1. **What are the foods that you turn to in sabotaging situations?** For some people it's sweets, for others it's fattening foods and for others it may be alcohol. 2. **What are the situations where you reach for those foods?** Is it a stressful day at work, an argument with a spouse or financial pressures? For some people there may be multiple associations, where one reaches for food in one circumstance but alcohol in another. 3. **Who are the people involved in these situations?** Perhaps a girlfriend loves to meet for dinner at all you can eat buffets. Are you agreeing to the restaurant choice? Maybe your husband has a dessert obsession. Are you using that as a perfect excuse for joining him?

Violet Smeltzer learned not to depend on food for comfort and lo. 40 pounds.

Confession #45, p. 180

Breaking the Self-Sabotage Cycle

Since self-sabotage is the result of unconscious eating associations that cause poor eating behaviors, **breaking the cycle requires you to create new associations that result in better behaviors.** The substitution of new behaviors must occur in any behavioral change. Take smoking cessation. Often an individual quits smoking but gains weight because they substituted eating food each time a cigarette craving occurred. This is an example of substituting one poor behavior for another. Alternatively, the individual could have done ten pushups or sit-ups or gone for a quick walk to get past a craving.

With food behaviors, one must take the "what" foods identified in self-sabotage and **choose alternative foods to eat or behaviors to follow when a craving arises**. For example, if an individual turns to ice cream when feeling blue, they could eat non-fat frozen yogurt in portion-controlled packages as an alternative. Even better would be finding a non-food substitution that involved activity. This would result in not eating the bad food choice and burning calories at the same time!

Situational triggers are a bit trickier because one can't control all external factors. A stressful day at work is going to happen, as is an argument with a significant other, family member or friend. Because it is the situations that trigger the eating, being aware of the associations and **having a clear plan regarding "what" you will do when the trigger occurs is what is necessary**. For instance, if after a bad day at work you have a tendency to sit down to a bottle of wine, cheese and crackers upon arriving home, instead keep an extra bag of exercise clothes in the car trunk and head directly to the fitness club or walking paths before going home.

Breaking "who-associations" often proves to be the most difficult; unless one moves to a new area and finds all new friends, "who-triggers" will remain. To overcome "who-triggers," **be assertive in choosing the activities that will be done with those who are triggers for sabotage**. When a friend suggests going to the buffet, propose a healthier alternative or simply decline. Secondly, communicate to these individuals that their assistance is needed for success. A true friend will understand and be supportive. If unwilling, perhaps it is time to re-evaluate friendships.

After losing weight many times, Judy Taylor lost 77 pounds by making a lifestyle change and now has a plan for whenever she falters.

Confession #46, p. 182

All of the suggestions for creating new behaviors with what, where and who eating associations require one to direct and control themselves, their environment and those around them. For many, this process is easier said than done. Lack of awareness and lack of trying, however, will never result in breaking the cycle and creating new behaviors.

Back in the Saddle...Again

When a woman relapses and gains some or all of her weight back she finds herself back in the early stages of behavioral change. Some will revert all the way back to pre-contemplation and remain in denial until another wake up call is delivered. Others will revert to contemplation ("I should . . . ") and still others only fall back to preparation ("I'm going to . . . ") The sooner an individual returns to the action stage, the greater the chances are for the next attempt to be successful.[24] The reasons for this are two-fold. First, the learning experiences gained from a failed attempt are fresher in the mind, allowing for a conscious change in strategy the next time. Second, assuming some behavioral change had taken place, it is easier to restart with a 10 or 20-pound re-gain than with a 50-pound regain; this is true both physically and emotionally.

To get back into action **re-start the process**; establish a S.M.A.R.T. goal and write out the compelling reasons why success is a must this time around; outline a nutrition and exercise plan; organize yourself with meal planning and food preparation; set up accountability and support systems with friends and family, get back to food journaling and step on the scale regularly, and; maintain control over external environments like social settings, dining out, and vacations. Most importantly, learn from your previous attempts, identify potentially dangerous situations and come up with alternative strategies.

---

[24] James O. Prochaska, John C. Norcross and Carlo C. DiClemente, Changing for Good (New York: Avon Books, 1994), p. 222-231.

Next, **know that there is no such thing as failure; there are only learning experiences!** If a child was learning a new skill and failed at the first attempt, no parent would allow them to quit. Instead, the parent would coach them on the skills and teachings needed to improve their performance and then give encouragement to keep trying. The expression "practice makes perfect" applies just as much to eating and exercise behaviors as it would any other skill. The only difference is that with adults the embarrassment of failure often overrides the sound advice that would be given to a child.

Joanne Breslin gained confidence and humility when she conquered her weight loss goal of losing over 30 pounds.

Confession #47, p. 185

There is one more piece needed to win the struggle to be thin <u>forever</u>: Humility. You must be humbled enough by the weight loss struggle that you know AND accept the reality that keeping your weight under control will be a life long battle. For many the struggle to keep weight off is no different than the struggle an alcoholic has to maintain sobriety. Where the difference lies, however, is that an alcoholic can maintain sobriety with abstinence. Unfortunately, abstinence from eating is not an option if one wants to live. This makes the struggle to be thin much more difficult in some ways than the struggle to remain sober. This in no way minimizes the challenge with sobriety nor does it provide the weight loss struggler with an excuse; it is simply the reality of the situation.

Many women who struggle with their weight have found the principles used in 12-step programs helpful in battling eating behaviors and food addictions. Knowing that the battle will be life-long, the 12-step approach helps them to maintain more control. Feeling in control provides a peace within. Some maintain perspective by reciting the serenity prayer daily. *God, grant me the serenity to accept the things I cannot change, the courage to change the things I can and the wisdom to know the difference.*[25]

After losing 35.2 pounds, Sandra Cosford is a changed woman on the outside and, more importantly, on the inside as well.

Confession #48, p. 188

---

[25] Reinhold Niebuhr, The Serenity Prayer (1926).

Chapter 9

Inspired

Inspired: "Outstanding or brilliant in a way or to a degree suggestive of divine inspiration."[26]

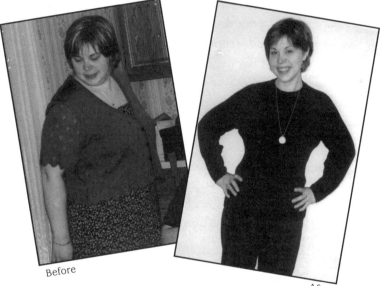

Before

After

Confession #49

Stacy Gilliom, Madison, WI
65 lbs. lost

I was diagnosed with a neurological disorder in the summer of 2000. I had no idea what it would mean for my life or the changes my body would undergo. I had always thought there'd be time to

[26] Webster's Dictionary

travel. I was overwhelmed and anxious. My weight was the last thing on my mind.

By the spring of 2003, I weighed 254 lbs. My activity level was already compromised and the added weight made it even harder to get around. My dreams of travel seemed impossible. I kept buying clothes in bigger sizes and consoling myself with food. I tried various workout programs, but nothing worked. Going to the gym was lonely. Just getting there was a victory, but there was no one to share it. Without a clear goal, it was easy to skip a couple weeks. Finally, I just gave up.

Upon a sudden inspiration, I took a job with Curves, convinced that if I was there all the time anyway I would work out more often. That much turned out to be true. I enjoyed the circuit and the ladies who came in to work out. But even though I was exercising regularly, I wasn't losing weight. I discovered that many of the members at Curves who were actually losing weight were also members of an independent weight loss organization such as Weight Watchers or Jenny Craig. I began to understand that weight loss and exercise are not mutually exclusive. They work in tandem.

I began to feel guilty when I signed up new members. Being a Curves employee tied my tongue. I couldn't tell these new members that exercise alone isn't enough. I wanted to tell them please don't expect to lose weight if they changed nothing else. Even though I was working out 3 to 4 times a week, I wasn't losing much weight either because I didn't understand nutrition. As a gym, Curves is a good one. But it felt wrong to allow women to believe that exercise alone would solve their weight dilemma. Why couldn't there be a place that combines the twin sisters of exercise and a healthy eating program?

Then one rainy summer day, I saw an ad for Healthy Inspirations. In the first picture there was a heavy-set woman who looked as tired and miserable as I felt. In the second picture, the same woman was smiling broadly with her hands on her much thinner hips. I went to my bathroom mirror and studied my reflection. I turned left, right, and then sucked in my stomach. It's no use, I sighed. I can't pretend anymore. I picked up the Healthy Inspirations ad again and looked at the confident, energetic woman in the picture. I looked at myself in the mirror again and thought, Why not? I picked up the phone and set an appointment.

I was greeted at the center by (a Lifestyle Consultant). Oh, great, I thought dismally, another perky woman with no idea how it feels to be this big. But I was wrong. On the way to the office, she pointed out her before and after pictures. I was amazed when I realized that the woman in the pictures was her! She had been through the program and it worked. We talked for almost an hour as she enthusiastically explained the various facets of Healthy Inspirations. Finally, I had found a program that combined exercise with a knowledge of nutrition. She had succeeded and I began to think that I could too. And succeed I did.

For 6 months, I met with consultants three times a week. Other women I met at the center were eager to share their success and congratulate me on mine. I started to look forward to working out. Going to the gym was no longer lonely. The circuit was almost always lively. I developed camaraderie with other women who were pursuing and achieving the same goals as me. I felt in control of my life for the first time since my diagnosis.

As the pounds decreased, I gained new energy and confidence. I learned not only what to eat, but why I was eating it. Knowledge of nutrition was something I craved but never got from other programs. Healthy Inspirations understands that weight loss is only the first step and that eating correctly for life is a vital part of success and health.

Seven months after I set foot in Healthy Inspirations, I boarded a flight to Europe. I had reached my goal of 185 pounds. Looking out the window of the plane, I thought about that fateful summer day. From those first shaky steps, I'd taken control of my weight, my illness, and my life. I listened to the hum of the engine and smiled. I thought about the new Healthy Inspirations ad I had taped on my bathroom mirror. This time, the confident woman in the picture with her hands on her much thinner hips was me.

Thank you Healthy Inspirations for your encouragement and your comprehensive program. You've helped me live a happier, healthier life!

What Stacy Didn't Know

Every few years Healthy Inspirations holds an essay contest for its members. Hundreds of applications have been submitted over the years. These stories, like the ones throughout this book, are incredible, heart-felt and inspiring. These women confess their struggles with weight and share their successes in the hopes of inspiring other women to want to change their lives too. When Stacy Gilliom submitted her essay in 2006, little did she know that she would be the grand prize winner of round trip airfare and accommodation to NY City and a $2,000 shopping spree and makeover! This is what she shares about her winning:

Epilogue:

After submitting my entry for the "Are You Inspired?" essay contest, my center-owner, surprised me with the news that I had won.

I was working out, having a grand time talking to some of the other women who were there, and taking a break from Monday. I was mid-sentence when a flash of color attracted my attention. (The center owner) came in carrying a bouquet of brightly colored balloons and beaming at me. I couldn't believe it. I had won! I had thought it was just staged drama when I saw people on TV jumping up and down when they won a big prize. It's not. I screamed and literally jumped out of my shoes. Sounds and sights became a blur, someone taking pictures, other members crowding around me, even my own voice sounded removed. I was in complete shock. All I could think was: Who am I going to call first?

I had no idea my story would touch so many women. I am not unique. I have no special will power, hidden talents, or determination that allowed me to succeed. I had simply had enough; enough of being tired, enough of people looking through me, enough of hiding in my home. Exercise alone wasn't the magic bullet I thought it would be. I needed both exercise and nutrition education. I was fortunate to find the solution in a program that is geared towards success for life, Healthy Inspirations. I succeeded. You can too.

Conclusion

Hopefully this book has provided you with divine inspiration! The goal was to give you the right information to guide you, but more importantly enough real life testimonials to inspire you to win your struggle to be thin. You aren't alone in your struggle and hopefully knowing that provides you with some solace. Ultimately, though, the inspiration to win your struggle must come from within. You hold the keys to freedom. You are in control of your destiny and you are the one who will reap the benefits and privileges of a healthier, slimmer, fitter life.

Additional inspiring success stories can be found in confessions #50-62 beginning on page 190 in appendix A.

Appendix A

Confessions

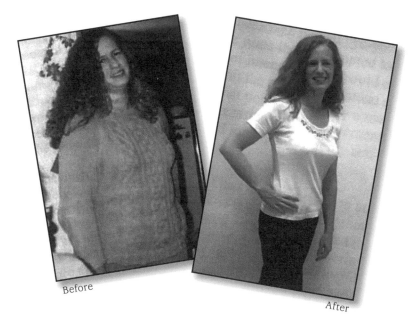

Before

After

Confession #2

Gretchen Williams, Camp Hill, PA
48.8 lbs. lost

Despite the fact that I have been relatively active throughout my life, I have continued to struggle with my weight. For this reason, I became a typical "yo-yo" dieter. I have lost count of the number of times throughout the years that I attempted to lose weight only to fail miserably. I would begin with the best of intentions and would even manage to lose some weight. Eventually, though, I would hit the inevitable plateau and become discouraged with my lack of progress. At that point it was only a matter of time until I would slip back into my poor eating habits, erasing any improvements I had made. This constant routine of failed attempts continued to chip away at my self-esteem, reinforcing the feeling that I was unable to succeed.

Although I continued to carry extra weight, I had always strived to attain a healthy lifestyle. I was faithfully working out five days a week, thinking that I was being proactive with my health. Then a routine blood screening revealed that my cholesterol level was 281! I knew I was facing a regimen of cholesterol lowering medication if I didn't manage to get my levels under control. If I was going to avoid medication, something had to change! It was time to stop trying to fight this battle alone. I had to face the fact that I needed help.

I chose Healthy Inspirations because of the friendly, inviting atmosphere and sensible eating plan. I particularly enjoyed the one-on-one coaching sessions offered through the Healthy Inspirations program. The staff at the Center offered the support I needed to stay focused. When I would experience a lull in my weight loss, they were always ready with encouraging words to remind me of the progress I had already made. They were more than just staff; they were my own personal support team. They were the friends I needed to help me face this challenge. That encouragement helped me through one plateau after another. I was beginning to think that I could really accomplish my goals this time!

In five short months, I lost nearly 50 pounds, reaching a goal that had eluded me throughout my many failed attempts in the past. I decreased my body fat percentage from 39% to 23%, lost a total of 33 overall inches and, most importantly, dropped my cholesterol level to a healthy 195! The good news doesn't stop there. There are more improvements. Improvements that can't be calculated with tape measures, scales, or even blood tests. I feel better about myself knowing that, with help, I was able to finally reach that goal that had eluded me for so long. It has been almost ten months since I reached my goal weight, and with the support of the staff at Healthy Inspirations, I have been able to maintain a healthy weight. I even did something a few months ago that I have never done before in my life… I cleaned out my closet and donated my "big clothes" to charity. This may seem like an uneventful, routine thing to do, but for me it was the final step. I wasn't making space in my closet; I was cleaning out all the self-doubt and low self-esteem that had been accumulating for so long. That was the point when I allowed myself to accept what I had accomplished, to allow myself to say, "I am not a failure. I can succeed!" I have my friends at Healthy Inspirations to thank for that!

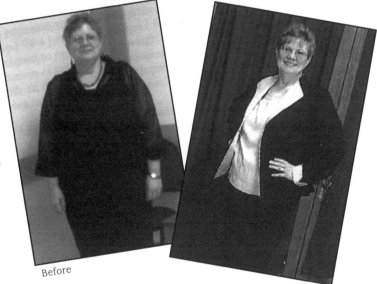

Before

After

Confession #3

Frances Leiter, Camp Hill, PA
44 lbs. lost

I was filled with despair before I learned about Healthy Inspirations. I was nearly 100 pounds overweight, my blood pressure was elevated, my knee was not recovering from surgery as expected, my feet and ankles pained me frequently and I had little self-esteem. I held out little hope for a job promotion and I felt I was an embarrassment to my husband, although he seemed resigned to my excessive weight. I couldn't generate much excitement about future retirement because of my history of continuous weight gain and the fear of becoming morbidly obese, along with all the associated health problems. The thought of by-pass surgery was frightening, and thankfully, my insurance carrier dropped coverage for it so I was unable to pursue it.

During my Healthy Inspirations consultation, I discovered that the program was not very different from my lifestyle and because of that I was concerned whether or not the program would work. However, in desperation, I enrolled in the program, hoping for a miracle. I was surprised by the quantity of food I was supposed to eat; evidently I had nearly killed my metabolism by trying to starve myself on my "healthy diet." My next surprise was that the scale actually started moving...downward!

Healthy Inspirations works! The eating plan is chemically and calorically balanced, making it an effective weight loss tool. It was relatively easy for me to follow and I did welcome the daily addition of fruit since I usually ate it only in season. The friendly counselors have been very encouraging and supportive, making it easy to stop by for the daily visits. They often offer suggestions and new recipes to make the plan more interesting and easier to stay on target. They told me how to maximize the benefit of my workout.

My weight loss has been fairly consistent and I have lost about 45 pounds. I did manage to land a new job, but it proved to be extremely stressful, thus my weight loss slowed down. I just returned to my former position and I am expecting to concentrate once more on following the eating plan diligently in hopes of resuming a weekly loss of 2 or more pounds.

The changes in my life have been most rewarding. I feel much better physically and emotionally. My knee has improved dramatically and I have been able to ditch my cane! I am much more agile too and I look forward to enjoying the outdoors more. My flower gardens have suffered since my surgery but I will be able to tend and enjoy them again. My doctor is happy with my weight loss and lowered blood pressure.

Perhaps the greatest reward though has been in my marriage. My self-esteem has improved dramatically and my husband is excited about my new image. We are planning retirement and I am eager to get out and explore the nature trails and wonders of this land, opportunities that I thought were lost due to my limited mobility, agility, endurance, and lack of interest. I now have hope that my "golden years" will be full of activity and health rather than filled with hopeless weight gain, poor health, and despair. Life now holds new interests and opportunities – all because of Healthy Inspirations.

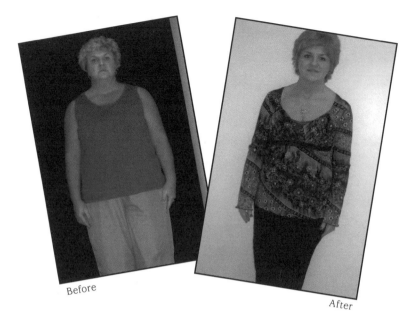

Before

After

Confession #4

Vanessa Morris, Fishersville, VA
60 lbs. lost

I began my journey with Healthy Inspirations because I was tired of being tired . . . I was an angry, overweight woman. I was not happy with anything in my life. When I looked in the mirror, I was disgusted with the way I looked. I felt fat and ugly. My solution for this feeling was to eat away my troubles and feelings, trying to find solace in food. This of course did not help matters, as I felt bad for overeating. The subsequent weight I added would then start the process all over again. I was caught in this vicious circle and could not see any way out. Then by chance I was reading my local newspaper and saw an advertisement for Healthy Inspirations. At first I was skeptical, because I think I have tried every diet known to man. After reading the article, I wrote down the website address and went online to look at the website. The more I read, the more I thought this might just work

and there might be a place for me at Healthy Inspirations. I called
the local office and made an appointment. I still had some doubts
about the program, that it would be like every other diet I have tried,
but I figured that I had nothing to lose but maybe some weight.

I arrived at my appointment with, what I must admit were, a little
more than a few butterflies. Then I walked in the door and I was
hooked. I have never felt more a part of something so quickly.
Healthy Inspirations has been like an extended family. The staff
members are always there for me with encouragement and advice
anytime I need them. If I miss a couple of days they call me and
make sure everything is okay and tell me that they are thinking
about me. The food plan was easy to follow and I never got hungry.
The supplements are awesome and I actually enjoy them.

I could not believe how fast the weight came off once I got started.
In the first month, I lost twenty pounds and fourteen inches. When I
measured, they gave me a piece of ribbon to show the inches as they
came off. To date I have lost sixty pounds and forty-seven inches. I
need to tell you that is a lot of ribbon. I am now free to shop in stores
and know they will have my size. The feeling of having that freedom
is beyond words. I am now a size fourteen and loving every minute
of it. I have not felt this good about myself in over twenty years.

The experience I have had with Healthy Inspirations has been nothing short of wonderful. I not only feel better and have energy I never
thought I would ever have again, but I truly love the way I look. I
feel so good about myself, and this has helped me with my relationship with my family. My daughter and I go shopping and do things
together we never have done.

In closing, I would just like to say that Healthy Inspirations has
changed my life in so many ways. I have learned not only how to live
a healthier life in the way that I eat and exercise, but I have learned
so many lessons about who I am and how my physical appearance
affects the way I approach so many aspects of my life.

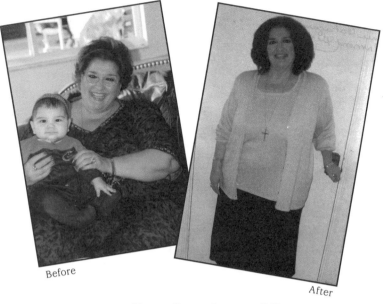

Before

After

Confession #5

Renee Gahagan, Ormond Beach, FL
101.5 lbs. lost

As a Human Services professional who has spent her entire life caring for people and advocating for the working poor who have fallen through the cracks, in one short year, I have become a person that I advocate for—I find what has happened to me mind blowing!

For over twenty years, I had a very successful career in development raising money for agencies geared to helping abused and abandoned children, rape victims, the developmentally disabled and the list goes on.

In one week in June of 2004 my life changed. My mom was diagnosed with Alzheimer's, I divorced, I was hit with hurricanes Charlie and Francis which added a $45,000 debt on my head because of no insurance, I lost my very secure job, and my son got married. Seeing him marrying his soul mate, a young lady whom we all love should have been a happy day for me and it was the most miserable day of my life. I was fat, out of shape and old! And we won't even discuss the plane ride and how I sat on the person's lap next to me because I didn't fit in the seat... the depression was too great. My weight blossomed to a staggering 367 lbs. and my health was declining. I didn't want to leave the house or see anyone. I refused to answer calls or emails from dear friends. I wanted to just die locked up in my house.

One day a friend knocked on my door and read me the riot act. She literally picked me up and forced me to come to Healthy Inspirations. I went kicking and screaming. Then another friend who realized my state of mind called to say that she would go with me to be my workout partner. This beautiful young woman was my inspiration to get back to what I used to look like when I tipped the scales at 135 lbs. and had a perfect 36-24-26 frame.

Today I weighed in 101.5 lbs. less and am continuing my journey. I have even started my own business, which was due to the encouragement of my cousin and friend. The business is taking baby steps in getting started, the same steps that it has taken me to get where I am today. Faith, commitment, determination and Healthy Inspirations have become my new vocabulary.

I have tried every diet plan known to man and not one ever taught me how to eat and why I was eating. I know that the key to my success is the workout regimen and the dieting which go along with the caring lifestyle consultants at Healthy Inspirations.

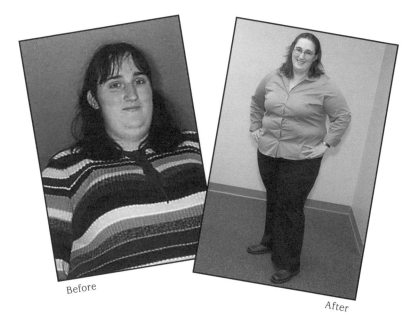

Before

After

Confession #7

Tara DeFranco, Lancaster, PA
30 lbs. lost

My journey to Healthy Inspirations' doorstep began when my father
became sick with cancer in 2004. Before he passed away, we had a
conversation that, "if there were no more conversations," we would
both be content with as a final conversation. I asked my father "Is
there anything you would change about me and the things I've done
in my life?" On the road of life, I had made mistakes and I wanted to
see how he felt about me. My father knew what I was getting at. He
lovingly reassured me that he was proud of me and my accomplishments in life. He only wished I took better care of myself.

I started to really think about that conversation with my father. I
had gained over 100 pounds when I was pregnant with my daughter
back in 2001. The weight never came off. I had tried numerous fad
diets and even went to a professional weight loss doctor. All of the

diets worked in the beginning, but the weight I took off would always creep back on. This led to my "I guess I'm meant to be fat" attitude.

When I first made the consultation appointment at Healthy Inspirations, I had my father on my mind, but I also had my own motivations. I wanted to be able to be more active with my daughter and I wanted to improve my lifestyle before the weight led to health issues that might eventually take me away from my family. I also wanted to lose the weight for myself so that I could feel better, look better, and have a better outlook on life. That's when I was finally motivated to start Healthy Inspirations.

There are many aspects of Healthy Inspirations that I enjoy. One part of the program I enjoy is that Healthy Inspirations is for women. Weight loss for me had always been private. I didn't want to exercise in a place where I felt like I was on display in front of everyone. Before joining, I had always felt like my weight loss battle was unique. My view changed once I started working out and some friendly conversation with some of the ladies made me realize that they were going through some of the same issues that I was. Now I look forward to my conversations with the other ladies because I feel supported and not alone.

Another aspect of Healthy Inspirations that I enjoy is how supportive and dedicated the staff is to my weight loss. I enjoy checking in instead of dreading it. The staff genuinely cares and relates to my weight loss struggle. They always offer suggestions on improvement and never judge if I have a slip-up in my diet.

There have been many great results from joining Healthy Inspirations. I am starting to appreciate foods that never entered my vocabulary before starting the program. When I go to the grocery store, I pick up products that are healthier better choices, rather than fatty foods or junk foods. Amazingly, I'm actually starting to enjoy those foods and make the decisions to eat them without even thinking about it or struggling with it.

Since joining Healthy Inspirations, I can actually say I have better self-esteem and I feel good about the healthy choices I make daily. I have much more energy since joining the program. I enjoy going to the gym and I can feel a change in my intensity with every workout.

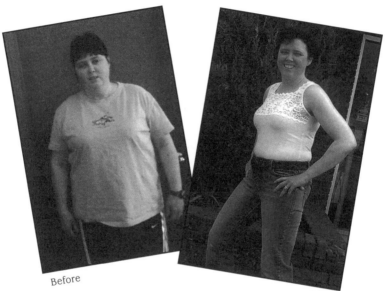

Before

After

Confession #8

Shelley Branconnier, Westerly, RI
60 lbs. lost

Have you ever looked in the mirror and said to yourself, "Wow, . . . I really need to lose some weight." Have you ever been so ashamed of your weight you actually bought men's clothing just because you could buy a smaller size? I mean for some crazy reason, a large in the men's section is much more appealing than an extra large in the women's. Well that's the position I was in when I walked through the door at Healthy Inspirations in Westerly, RI August 17, 2005.

At 5'3", I weighed a depressing 200 pounds. I could blame it on the immune suppressing drugs I take every day to treat my lupus. What about the joint pain, fibromyalgia or chronic fatigue? Lupus is quite skilled at making you feel as if you have just run a twenty mile marathon when all you really did was walk from the couch to the snack cupboard. Maybe it's the cotri-steroids I use to keep my asthma under control. I also take prednisone every day, which happens to be the grandmother of weight gain. I had a million excuses and I used them all for a long time. I wasn't living life to the fullest because of my weight. I couldn't even walk up a flight of stairs without needing oxygen. I did nothing but watch as the numbers on the scale continued to rise. I was depressed and extremely unhappy with myself. Excuses came easily and it wasn't difficult to beat myself up. The hard part was finding the motivation to change it. Self-hatred, low self esteem and depression had a tight grip. It was time to put an end to all these excuses. I decided to challenge myself and accept responsibility for my own weight gain. I had found comfort in telling myself "you will never be thin, you take too many medications, you are just too sick to change it." But wearing men's clothing? When had I accepted that? Were diabetes and high blood pressure just part of getting older? How did I let it get so out of control? I had to take charge of my health and my life. Now all I needed was motivation. I knew I had to make some big changes. Healthy Inspirations gave me the knowledge and support to make it happen. I now have a new outlook on food, a new outlook on me, and a brand new outlook on life. I finally took responsibility for me. Ownership, it worked and it feels good.

The program is really pretty simple, eat healthy and exercise for life. It's not a diet, those are only temporary. This is about commitment, accountability, knowledge, encouragement and an amazing support system. Food is everywhere and weight loss is a long road, but the lifestyle counselors are willing to walk with me every step of the way. They know it's not easy. It's good days and bad; it's ups and downs; it's highs and lows; but it is always about me. They assist me in setting goals, and work hard to ensure I reach them. They know my personality and understand my issues with food. They care, and I know it. Support makes all the difference between success and failure, and success feels good.

In seven months I have lost 60 pounds and 69.5 inches. I went from a size 18 to a size 6. My confidence is climbing every day. For the first time in years I actually feel good about myself. I am a new person and the changes in my life are indescribable. I joined Healthy Inspirations to lose weight, but I've gained so much more. The lessons I've learned will be with me for the rest of my life. I have dedicated, caring and supportive friends. I mean hey, cheesecake happens. There is a support system out there for those of us who can't do it alone.

It has been the journey of a lifetime, and I have learned so much more than I could ever have imagined…. I actually know how to love myself. Wow, it really is all about me.

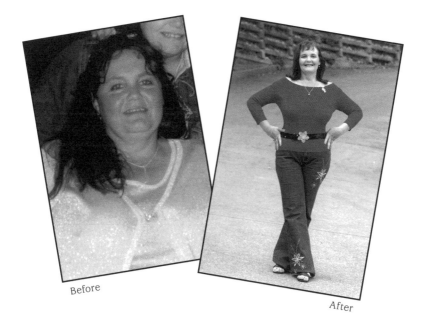

Before

After

Confession #9

Jennene Kirby, Palm Beach, Australia
100.8 lbs. lost

At 41 years of age I weighed 116.5 kilos (256 lbs.) and was a size 26. The weight was threatening my health and my doctor told me, "Lose weight or you could be in a wheelchair by the time you're 50." Even with that kind of ultimatum coming from a medical professional, it took my staying two months in a hospice-like hospital for me to realize he was telling me the truth!

When I finally made my way to Healthy Inspirations, I could barely walk into the Center because of chronic back problems and heavy medication. At first I thought I couldn't even lose 10 kilos (22 lbs.). All I could do was take one day at a time. One year later and I have lost 100 lbs. and gone from a size 26 to nearly a size 12 and my doctor has reduced my medication!

I know it's an old cliché, but if I can do it, anyone can. No one ever said losing weight was easy and it's not… But when you believe in yourself it is possible. Of course you have your ups and downs… I cried when I put on even just a bit of weight. But I always try to turn a negative into a positive with small incentives like trying to match the clothes sizes of my top and bottom. If I miss a workout, I don't feel guilty; I just take one day at a time and say to myself "today's the day and I have to do it," so I just do.

I definitely have new habits for life because now I understand how to eat healthily. Every day I know how much starch, protein, fruit, vegetables and dairy I need so I can even eat out and I know what to order so it's easy. More importantly, my sons are eating better too because they eat what's in the cupboard and it's all healthy. Ironically, now when I go in to see my doctor I check on how he is doing with losing the 10 kilos (22 lbs.) he needs to and I help keep him on track! Healthy Inspirations gave me a fresh start.

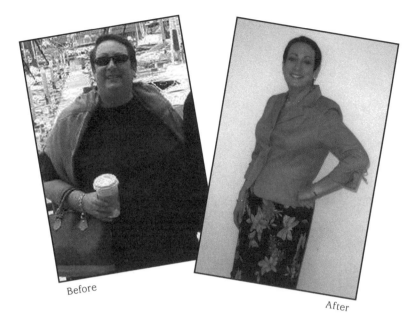

Before

After

Confession #11

Shelli Janoff, St. Petersburg, FL
122 lbs. lost

I joined Healthy Inspirations in late January 2005. At the time, I weighed 293 pounds. I had been overweight for more than fifteen years, and at this point I was seriously considering bariatric surgery because I didn't think I could ever lose all of the excess weight on my own. But luckily for me, when I went for a surgical evaluation the doctor told me I had to try one more time to lose weight before he would agree to operate. A friend at work told me about the Healthy Inspirations program, and I decided to sign up.

I was at a point in my life where my deteriorating health was a big concern. I was on the verge of becoming diabetic; my blood pressure was so high I had to take three different medications to control it; I was so obese I could hardly walk. My knees, hips and feet ached all of the time. I was absolutely miserable. I was truly convinced I would die before age 65.

The program appealed to me because both the diet counseling and exercise take place in the same location. The eating plan appeared to be a very healthy one, and the idea that I would have to sign a contract that included one year of maintenance after reaching my weight loss goal was very attractive. I've lost weight before but never been able to keep it off; this time I knew I wouldn't be on my own once I got to my desired weight. I also knew that the staff at the Center would not let me just give up, and would be there for moral support and to give me nutritional counseling when I hit a plateau or had difficulty sticking with the plan.

It's now March 18, 2006 and I weigh 172 pounds. Due to the benefits of the weight training machines, I can wear a size twelve in clothing. I feel and look like an entirely different person. All of the people who know me say I'm an inspiration to them to lose weight and develop a healthy lifestyle. At age fifty-five, I'm the happiest I've ever been in my life. I still have about forty pounds to go, but I know I can do it following the Healthy Inspirations eating plan and continuing my exercise regimen. I don't think I'll ever go back to eating the kinds of things and the quantity of food I used to eat. Now I enjoy the taste of food without salt, and I no longer tolerate foods high in fat. I feel so much better physically than I did before, it's just amazing. The staff at Healthy Inspirations . . . are wonderful, and have worked with me through rough spots and have celebrated with me as I lost 122 pounds. They feel just as good about my progress as I do.

My cholesterol, blood sugar and blood pressure have come down to the normal range and my doctor is thrilled. I'm not only a normal weight (soon to be at my ideal BMI [Body Mass Index]), but I can go places and do things I hadn't done for the last fifteen years. I'm a true believer in the Healthy Inspirations program, and have recommended it to anyone who asks me about my weight loss. In fact, a number of people at work have joined the program after talking to me about it. I look forward to being a healthy, active senior citizen someday, all because of Healthy Inspirations.

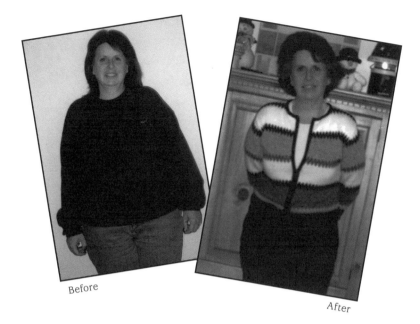

Before

After

Confession #12

Anne Marie Koohy, Middletown, RI
49.8 lbs. lost

I've always been on the chunky side most of my life. Even as a kid growing up, I always wondered what it would be like to be thin. I saw the advertisement in the local paper, looking for volunteers to do a weight loss study. It was time for me to make a choice, so I got up the nerve and with my husband's encouragement, went to a seminar. Talk about being scared, a room filled with about 100 women and I knew none of them but finally I could say, "Okay, I'm not alone."

When I went into the Middletown site, and met the staff, I felt comfortable with them. I knew then and there this was the place to be. I did get picked as part of the study and went forward with the program. I look back now and even if I wasn't picked, I do sincerely believe I would have stayed! I did it for me and I am worth it.

What was most important to me was the one on one coaching from the staff. They kept you focused and on track with good eating habits, exercise and breaking bad routines. The staff got me to rethink how and when to eat and how to work that into my job. I have a lot of stress at my job and when I have stress I eat. The staff at Healthy Inspirations showed me the good stuff to have and how to control what I was consuming.

Exercise was always difficult for me because I always made excuses why I couldn't do it. The staff made it fun and rewarding. I even got my husband to walk with me. That was a chore in itself.

One of the nice things I can say is that I got to meet different people, all aiming for the same goal and cheering each other on. If I missed a day or two, one of the staff members would call to make sure everything was okay. It was that personal touch, that feeling of belonging that got me over the tough times.

The results I experienced are grand. I am amazed that I have lost, 49.8 pounds, 9% body fat and a total of 46.75 inches. I have never felt as good as I do now. My lifestyle has changed for the better.

My self-esteem has risen and I feel great about who I am and now I enjoy being out and meeting new people. I really feel good about myself. My appearance has changed totally, inside and out. I feel that I can run circles around everyone.

Next to meeting my husband, this was the best choice I have made in my life. Thank you Healthy Inspirations for giving me my life back and enjoying the time I have to spend with family.

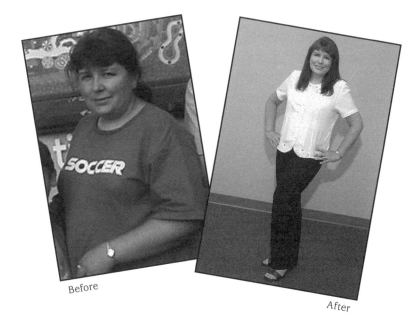

Before

After

Confession #13

Tara Faro, Lancaster, PA
30 lbs. lost

(I was) out of control, depressed, tired and scared. After struggling with my weight for years, I'd gotten to the point where it seemed easier to ignore it...food was a comfort, and I was in a cycle of eating when I was depressed, anxious or mad. Why give up the foods I like when it was so easy and enjoyable to eat as I pleased?

At 41 years old and 60 lbs. overweight, I knew I wouldn't be able to avoid high blood pressure, joint aches, high cholesterol, diabetes or heart problems much longer. Eating poorly and not exercising is guaranteed to lead to these problems – I knew that.

I wanted more time to spend with my sons. We stopped taking vacations because I kept thinking, "We'll go to Florida when I can fit into my old clothes, when I won't be too tired to walk up the stairs, when I'll look okay for pictures or videos". Later was turning into never.

I tried to exercise and keep track of what I ate, but it was inconsistent. Most of the foods I chose were too high in starches and sugar, so I wasn't losing weight; instead I was left feeling hungry. Sometimes I ate too much at one meal, just to gain back the pound that had taken days to lose. I'd get discouraged and give up. I was taking two steps forward and one backwards, and never getting anywhere.

Then last December I read an ad for Healthy Inspirations featuring 7 women who lost a total of 284 lbs. I looked at their pictures and thought if these women could be successful, then maybe I could be too.

I was nervous when I called to make an appointment, but when I first walked into Healthy Inspirations, I relaxed. There was a bio of the Lifestyle Consultants with their inspiring weight loss successes. It helped to know that they had struggled with weight loss and understood the challenges.

They asked me, "On a scale of 1 to 10, how willing are you to commit?" I replied "8 or 9"; I knew I'd have days when I wouldn't be perfect.

The program sounded ideal. They gave me a meal plan that's sensible but flexible. I met other women like me, of different ages and sizes. The exercise circuit helped to tone and rebuild my muscles. Knowing that three times a week I meet with the counselors to review my eating has kept me on track. They've helped to guide me and give me advice on days when I stumble. Healthy Inspirations offers snack bars that are more nutritious than other protein bars and help me get over any cravings. Special monthly meetings and seminars offer continuous support.

At times when I struggle with a decision of what to eat, I remember the commitment I made and the people that are pulling for me.

We all have a story to tell. Many of us struggle with the same issues and feelings of helplessness with weight loss. Whether it's 10 lbs. or 100+, it all begins in the same place – a food plan you can follow and live with everyday, an exercise plan that allows you to start slowly and build up strength, plus support from women who have been in your place.

So far, I've lost 30 lbs. in 15 weeks. Other positive changes are I've dropped two pant sizes, I have more energy, I'm less depressed and most importantly, I feel in control again. I'm not at my goal yet, but I have no doubt I can be successful for a lifetime.

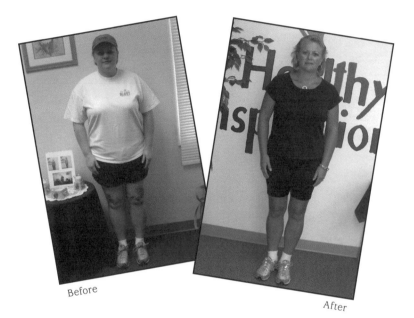

Before

After

Confession #14

Renee St. Clair, Forest VA
44.5 lbs. lost

My story begins 24 years ago – as a college freshman, I gained the "freshman 15" along with an additional 20. With an athletic and healthy background, this was a very depressing state to be in. Fast forward to one month ago, February 2006…after gaining and losing the same 20-30 pounds for 24 years, I decided to take charge of my life.

Following a financial and emotional crash when our new family business failed last year, I packed on 30 pounds in just over a year.

Always a stress eater, I now felt unattractive, under-appreciated, tired and unhealthy. A positive self-esteem was non-existent, and I could barely wait to take a nap after waking from a night's sleep. As a mother of two active boys, 2 ½ and almost 6, I knew I needed to do something to take care of myself, but the eye-opening call from my doctor announcing a cholesterol concern, really got me going. At 42, I knew that with a family history of diabetes, heart disease and cancer, that I would need to take charge of my health or I would never see my young children grow up to be adults.

After remembering the success of two good friends with the Healthy Inspirations life-changing plan, I thought it might be a good option for me. When I researched the plan, I knew there was no way I would slim down, since there was way too much food listed per day. What? Starches, fat, fruit and dairy? There's no catch for it? No way! After my Quick Start, and already 5 lbs. towards my goal, I could barely believe it could work so easily! I have had no cravings, because my body is fueled with a good balance of nutrients. With the balance of foods each day, and the watchful and encouraging staff, I have "melted" off 15 lbs. in just over 3 ½ weeks! I am halfway to my goal of 30 lbs. off, and it has been less than a month!

I am feeling healthier, and better than I have in years! I now have "pep in my step" that I wasn't sure I would ever feel again. There is just no stopping me now! I have my goals in sight, and with very little effort, my dream of feeling and looking good by this summer is very attainable! I finally feel good about myself, and this feeling of achievement is as important to me as the physical changes. I am not feeling like a "fat" person in a smaller shell, like I have in the past when I lost weight. I am sure that it is because it is a life change for me, and I know that my whole family is happier for my choices. I can't wait for this summer, and bathing suit weather. I never thought I would be excited to wear a swimsuit, but I will be proud to "strut my stuff" this summer!

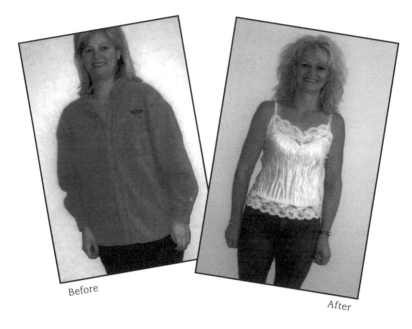

Before

After

Confession #15

Rose Flitz, Madison, WI
50 lbs. lost

For the past several years, I struggled so much with my weight and was always trying to lose the last ten pounds. After gaining fifteen pounds over the holidays in 2004, I decided that I was not going to turn forty and be forty pounds overweight. So I talked to my husband and I called Healthy Inspirations. That was the beginning of a life changing experience for me.

I met with the staff of Healthy Inspirations and began to meet some of the most kind, motivating people I have ever met. Every time I come into the Center, I feel like I have a group of cheerleaders there to cheer me on. Even when I come in and I have deviated from the plan, they motivate me and help me to get through the difficult times.

Since my start date of January 5, 2005, my life has changed in ways I really didn't expect. The original goal that I set for myself I have surpassed by seventeen pounds. I have reached a weight that is lower and healthier than any weight I have been. I have lost fifty pounds and five sizes. I now look at exercise as MY time for myself. Instead of an inconvenience, it is an enjoyment. I now need the time I take every week to walk/run and work out at the Center to just be me with no phones ringing and no interruptions.

Physically, I feel better than I ever have in my life. On my 40th birthday last year, I was in better shape and weighed less than I have my entire adult life. My blood pressure is the lowest it has ever been. I am wearing sizes that I still can't believe fit me! I love all the fun fashions I can wear now that I never could before. I will turn forty-one this year and so far I am maintaining my weight. I continue to go to the Center and work out three to four days a week; it has truly become a part of my life.

I am amazed at the difference in the way I cook now. Everything is so much healthier and it tastes great! As a result of my success my husband has been inspired and lost fifty pounds as well! I am a salon owner/stylist and have inspired many clients to join Healthy Inspirations to lose weight and live their best life as well.

Mentally, I'm happier with who I am and am more comfortable in my own skin than ever before. I know I did the work but I also know that I could not have done it without the unending support of my loving husband and of course without the guidance and support of my friends at Healthy Inspirations.

I would like to thank everyone at Healthy Inspirations, Madison, Wisconsin for always making me see that I could do it. I would also like to thank them for the constant support and "cheerleading". Every one of the people at the Center is fabulous and they are changing lives every day in many ways. I can never thank them enough!

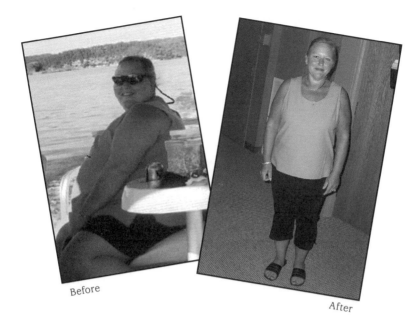

Before

After

Confession #16

Christina Escalona, Rogers, AR
100+ lbs. lost

I have been overweight for as long as I can remember. I began dieting in my elementary years and was wearing a size 20 by high school.
Though I was already obese, I managed to gain an additional 60
pounds with the birth of my daughter that I was never able to lose.

In October of 2003 I attended a team meeting in Arizona with the
company I work for. One of our "team building" activities was to ride
horses through a barrel course. It took four cowboys (and a lot of
effort) to get me on my horse, which was a very embarrassing ordeal.
After completing the ride the cowboys struggled to help me get off
my horse, only to learn that the nightmare was not over. I had to get
back on another horse to herd cattle! By the time I was done I was
humiliated and in tears. This was the final straw.

When I returned home I went to my doctor to inquire about having gastric bypass surgery. Two of my sisters had already had this surgery but my doctor had concerns about it and would not give me a referral. A few days later I was listening to the radio and I heard an advertisement for a Healthy Inspirations meeting that caught my attention. I decided to attend that meeting where I was able to learn about the Health Inspirations program. I was also able to see and hear from local ladies who had already experienced success on the program. While I had already tried many other programs (Nutrisystem, Jenny Craig, Optifast, Weight Watchers) over the years, I decided to try one more time.

I started the Healthy Inspirations program in November 2003 right after having knee surgery. I needed to lose over 100 pounds, which was a little overwhelming, but the support of the staff plus the fact that I had to weigh-in three times a week helped keep me on track. Starting right before the holiday season was also a challenge, but Healthy Inspirations gave me the additional support and motivation I needed to help me get through the holidays without cheating.

So far I have lost over 100 lbs. and am now hooked on exercise. When I started I could not walk up my driveway. Now I go to Spinning classes 3-4 times a week and walk 5-8 "hilly" miles a day. I have made so many changes in my lifestyle; it is as if I am a completely different person. I can now buy clothes anywhere I choose and have the luxury of knowing that even on an airplane, my seat belt will fit!

Healthy Inspirations has made such a HUGE difference to me and I am so thankful to them for helping me feel "normal" for the first time in my life.

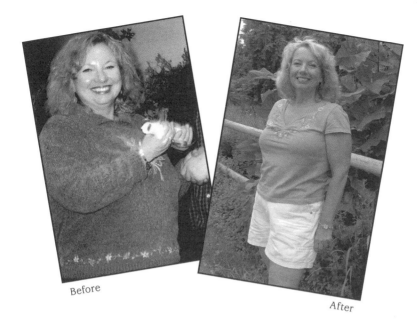

Before

After

Confession #18

Denise Huffman, Cranston, RI
53 lbs. lost

From the time I was a child, I always had a weight problem. My dad was a lover of ice cream, so almost every night we would sit together and enjoy each other's company over a bowl. He also loved soda, which was a staple in my house; however we did not share that common love. My drink of choice was fruit juice and being a lot more expensive, my father still indulged me figuring they were at least "good for me." Now as an adult, I know they are loaded with calories and lots of sugars. Pasta was also a big staple in our house and lord only knows all the fresh bakery breads, rolls and pastry my dad brought home to us. Needless to say, I acquired a fierce appetite for the highest calorie foods.

I went on diets as a teenager practically starving myself to "fit in" with the other girls but as soon as I got married and had a child it was the beginning of the end. My weight boomeranged back and forth over and over again from size 7 to size 20. I tried Weight Watchers, Jenny Craig, fad diets such as Atkins, low carbs but everything became a bigger and bigger bandage for all my wounded body parts. They call it yo-yo diets but that is too broad and kind. What it does, or should I say did, was cause high blood pressure, bad thyroid, lack of energy and malaise.

I found out about Healthy Inspirations from a very good friend of mine who also shared similar problems. I thought, "Well it can't hurt, exercise and weight loss in one place sounds like a good idea!" So I joined in December and started slow but by January I was exercising at least 3 or 4 days a week. Now I have lost 53 pounds, several inches and am now obsessed with exercise because it is actually fun! There are Group Power classes as well as circuit exercising along with Synergie (cellulite treatments), a relaxation chair, a Tone and Talk class, all of which I participate in and it is never boring. I have now learned how to eat, when to eat certain foods and really am never hungry. It has been an inspiration and joy to meet all the great people at the Center and how everyone helps one another.

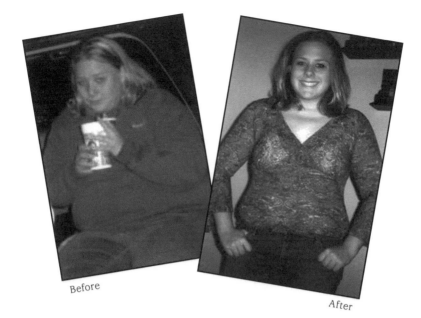

Before

After

Confession #19

Stacey Pues, Ormond Beach, FL
80 lbs. lost

I recently graduated from Appalachian State University and a
college education was not all I gained in my four years in North
Carolina. I was around fifty pounds overweight when I started my
freshman year in 2001 and managed to gain an additional eighty
pounds. In my four-year journey, I watched my friends do considerable damage to their bodies trying to lose weight; bulimia, anorexia
and addiction to diet pills made me lose hope of battling obesity in a
healthy way.

I attempted to lose weight by taking pills, participating in fad diets,
weight loss programs, therapy and exercise. However, I could never
find a winning combination. I would see myself getting bigger and
bigger and farther away from caring. The depression of being obese
would lead to an instant gratification process of drinking alcohol

and then indulging in unwholesome eating and eventually end up gaining more weight. My desire to look good in a pair of jeans was moving quickly towards a desperate need for help to improve my physical condition for health reasons.

I first came into Healthy Inspirations during my last spring break in March 2005. I was convinced the program would work. The words of two to three pounds a week guaranteed weight loss echoed in my mind for five months; I promised myself I would come back in August after I graduated.

When I finally moved down to Daytona Beach to pursue my dream of working for NASCAR, I decided I would try to lose the weight on my own because, like everyone else just finishing school, I was broke. For three weeks straight I ate very light and walked five miles every day. I got on the scale after those three weeks and I had lost a little under a pound. I was devastated.

I decided that that I would not wait any longer. So on August 19th, 2005, I decided to take a step to try to change my life. I went down to Healthy Inspirations and signed up. After the first week on the program I had lost seven pounds, which was extremely captivating because I was eating a lot, and had only exercised three times that week!

After the first month I was down twenty pounds.[27] It felt so good to finally succeed losing weight a healthy way. And now seven months later, I am down almost 80 lbs. My friends are so impressed that I have done it with a good diet and exercise they say I am an inspiration to them. My co-workers at the speedway also notice the change in my body and call me skinny!

My favorite part about the program and the most essential is the guidance and individualized support from the coaches. Without them, this program would not be possible. I can tell by the looks on their faces how proud of me they are and that leads me to be proud of myself. I feel like I have joined a family and that this program is what really changed my life. Through their continuing support, I have learned that eating until exploding is not rewarding and I

---

[27] A weight loss of this amount in one month is not typical.

finally feel for the first time in my life that I am eating to live rather than living to eat.

I am extremely confident with Healthy Inspirations I will be able to lose the rest of my weight, keep it off, and most importantly GAIN self-esteem and become the confident, sexy businesswoman that I have been longing to become! Thank you Healthy Inspirations!

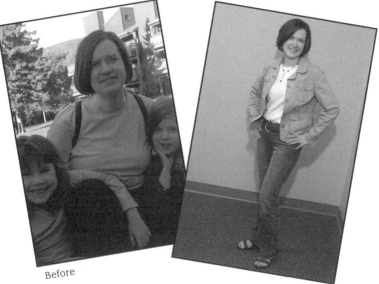

Before

After

Confession #20

Stacey Kubis, Lancaster, PA
23 lbs. lost

Healthy Inspirations provided me with more than just a weight-loss plan. I have almost always been at least 10 pounds over my "ideal" weight, but last year I underwent kidney surgery and quickly gained 10 more pounds while I was recovering. The holidays were then upon me and my 35th birthday was rapidly approaching. Being a stay-at-home-mom to two young, impressionable girls (ages 7 and 5), I decided it was time to lose the extra weight. More importantly, I needed to be a positive role model for my children and teach them how to eat right and make physical activity a priority. Healthy Inspirations gave me the tools to achieve both of my goals, losing the extra weight and modeling a healthy lifestyle through good food choices and a commitment to exercise.

The Healthy Inspirations program has so many positive attributes. The eating plan is easy to follow and the results are immediate and sustainable. I know I am making good food choices, and the program has taught my family which foods are best. For example, after listening to the CD on the benefits of soy, my younger daughter, who was four at the time, blurted out during lunch that she wanted soy milk because "soy is good for you!" Secondly, the Healthy Inspirations center is such a welcoming place. Both the staff and other program participants are unrelenting in their support. The staff are knowledgeable and have battled weight issues themselves. The other women in the program share tips, struggles, and encouragement. There are book clubs, special seminars, and additional services such as Synergie, the infrared sauna, and massage chair to complement the program. The supplements taste great and are affordable. Furthermore, Healthy Inspirations includes an exercise regime, a key to losing weight and keeping it off! The resistance circuit, while easing you into an exercise routine, builds lean muscle so you burn more calories. Healthy Inspirations offers a complete package – an easy to follow and effective weight-loss plan and an encouraging, educational environment.

Healthy Inspirations gave me the tools to meet my goals. I lost 23 pounds and many, many inches. I went from a size 10 petite to a size 4 petite. My hydration ratio increased 7% to 57%! My BMI, now solidly in the healthy range, dropped 4 points. My self confidence is at an all-time high. I am in great physical shape. I can now easily run 6 miles. But more importantly, my family is making healthy choices. We eat more fruits, vegetables, fish, soy, and complex carbohydrates. We visit the gym almost daily. I know my girls will continue to eat right and exercise regularly. They see me do it and are aware of the positive impact of a healthy lifestyle.

Thanks to Healthy Inspirations I have become the role model I want to be for my children, and we are inspired to be healthy together!

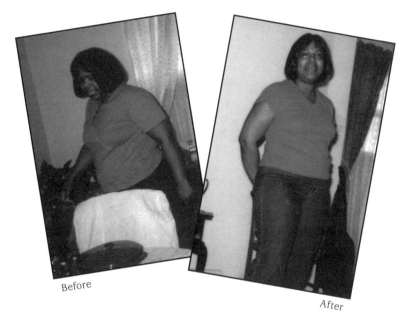

Before

After

Confession #21

Deborah Hunter, Springfield, PA
33 lbs. lost

My name is Deborah Hunter. I have tried many different diets without success. It seemed that after each failed diet I ended up even heavier than I was before starting the diet. One day while watching TV, I heard a man say that most people do not have a blood pressure problem but they have a weight problem. The man said most high blood pressure is caused by obesity. I looked up the guidelines for obesity and found that I fit that description.

Being overweight turned shopping, one of my favorite pastimes, into torture. At size twenty in women's, it became very difficult to find anything that I liked. It got to the point that I just would not buy anything for myself. The only clothes I had were given to me by my mother. A lot of them I did not really like but I just wore them because I felt that I would not find anything I liked anyway, so it did not matter.

One of my co-workers began to lose weight noticeably. I asked and she told me she had been going to Healthy Inspirations. Since I was tired of getting short of breath going up and down stairs and just tired of being tired in general, I decided to go.

I was a little nervous about going. I did not want to spend more money to fail again. The personnel at Healthy Inspirations were very encouraging and made me feel that I could definitely accomplish my desired weight loss goal. . . .

I like the fact that the program includes diet and exercise instruction. There are personal trainers there that help you design an exercise program for you. For instance, there were a couple of things I could not do and I was given alternatives that would work the same muscles. I had recently been told that I had osteopenia and I needed an exercise program that incorporated weight training. This was available for me at Healthy Inspirations.

Even though I am not at my goal yet, I have not given up and I plan to continue until I reach it. At this point, I am 50% to my goal but I am no longer wearing men's sizes. I can actually go out and find an outfit that I like. Shopping for clothes is no longer the chore it had been. I have not bought a lot at this time because I still have weight to lose, but for the first time in years I can see a light at the end of the tunnel as far as my weight is concerned.

Not only has my size gone down, but also my energy has gone up. I still remember the first time I went up the stairs and I looked down and couldn't believe how good I felt. I actually ran up and down a couple of times just to see if it was my imagination. Also, I had been on blood pressure medicine for several years, at this point I am on half the blood pressure medication I was on a year ago and my doctor thinks that as I lose weight I may eventually be able to get off the medication completely.

Healthy Inspirations has helped me to become an inspiration to others.

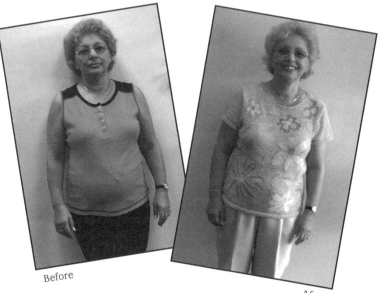

Before

After

Confession #22

Shoshana Haas, Jacksonville, FL
16 lbs. lost

My first encounter with Healthy Inspirations took place at a health expo. Since I am very wellness-oriented, the name of the organization caught my attention. The people who were representing the company were very slim and apparently in quite good health. I knew that their appearance was the one that I wished to have for myself.

The image that they portrayed was very inspiring to me, so my commitment was instantly born. I made an appointment and signed up immediately.

Like so many others, I have tried numerous other plans to lose weight, and they were frequently successful. However, my "wins" were always temporary, as unfortunately, I always managed to "find" all that I had lost.

From the beginning with Healthy Inspirations, I felt as though I was in a university-type environment where I was taught how, what and even when to eat and how to combine (or not) the intake of certain foods.

Also, I was given excellent instruction and demonstration in the use of the wide variety of exercise equipment. The nutritional counseling and exercise demonstrations were all carefully monitored and supervised by the capable and knowledgeable coach who worked with me during every session. Healthy Inspirations is definitely goal-oriented, so there were certain expectations for each and every exercise period in which I have participated.

In addition to instruction in proper eating habits and proper exercise, I was also constantly reminded that we must be diligent about keeping our bodies well hydrated, as water is one of the most important elements of all living things.

I quickly realized that in order for this great program to work well for me, there was no choice but to make a total commitment to it. Attending these sessions become an inspiration (no pun intended) for me and NOTHING has been allowed to interfere with my intention. I was – and still do - maintain this obsession with keeping my appointments three times each and every week. Obviously, I have been inspired and committed 100%. I have always felt much better after the completion of my exercise routine.

Since beginning my individualized program with Healthy Inspirations over fifteen months ago, I have met many interesting people and created new friendships with people who share a passion for good health. The staff is always very friendly and helpful and the environment is one that provides an atmosphere of a "can do" attitude.

Thus far, I have "shed" sixteen pounds and ten inches and have no doubt that I will eventually reach my goal of twenty pounds. There are numerous women in this program who have lost considerably more weight than that, however. I feel so much better, both physically and mentally and I know that I project this image to others in my environment. The feedback that I receive is that I look young and radiant. This image has inspired other women at my workplace to follow my lead and sign up with Healthy Inspirations to improve their own lives and sense of well being. Not surprisingly, they too are now experiencing results similar to mine,

The location and hours of operation are very convenient for me, the cost is very affordable and the facility is always clean. For these reasons, as well as all of the above, I am very pleased that I joined Healthy Inspirations. I hope that this testimonial will serve to inspire other women towards better health.

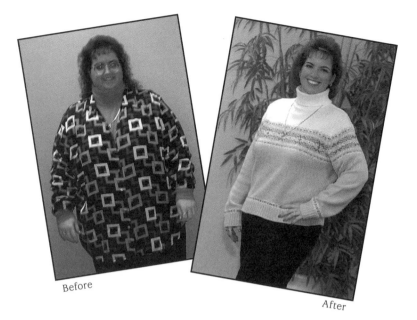

Before

After

Confession #24

LeAnn Varano, Lancaster, PA
109.5 lbs. lost

I joined Healthy Inspirations in January 2005 because I didn't like what I saw when I'd look in the mirror. My back hurt, I had trouble with my knees, and I just wasn't happy with ME. I decided it was time to do something so I made a phone call to set up an appointment to find out what this was all about.

After making the commitment to go through with the program, I had my Program Explanation. When I got home, I was so overwhelmed that I wasn't sure I could do this! The plan and all the "rules", the journaling, the exercise, losing my snacks and "junk" food – it was a LOT to comprehend. After only a few weeks, I had things under control and was able to put meals together with more confidence that I was well on my way to eating and being much healthier.

What I like most about the program is the amount of support from not only the staff, but also other women clients who are working toward a goal of their own. There's camaraderie and friendships to be formed when you're working out with others who are in the same program. Recipe swapping and sharing ideas for meals helps everyone change things up so it's not the same thing all the time. I had a slow start with only losing 1-1/2 pounds on Quick Start so I knew it would be an up hill battle for me. Setting a goal of losing 100 lbs. was one I wasn't so sure I'd be able to accomplish but I was going to give it all I had!

Fifteen months later, I'm down 109-1/2 pounds and have lost over 60 inches off my body. I have no more back pain, my knees are better, I have more self esteem, and much improved muscle tone. Not to mention the more nutritionally balanced eating and over all healthier body. I feel AND look better than I ever have before and I hope my success will help others to see the program really works if the desire and discipline is there to make it work!

All the journaling, being accountable for everything I eat, the support, and overwhelming desire to reach my goal has transformed my mind into wanting a healthier lifestyle. I have more energy and don't like to sit around. I like to stay busy and I'm enjoying life a LOT more. Thank you Healthy Inspirations for giving me the information and the tools I needed to reach my goal and make me a healthier person!

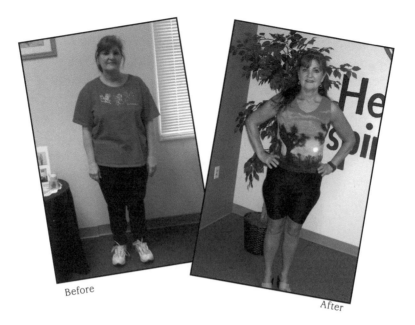

Before

After

Confession #25

Brenda Robertson, Forest, VA
32 lbs. lost

The way I choose to approach my life used to be complicated, but not anymore.

I was so focused on making sure that everyone else's needs were met that I neglected my own. I put my weight concerns on the back burner. As my weight kept climbing, I realized I had to set limits and make myself and my health a priority. I got tired of hearing my loved ones telling me I was getting "fat" especially with my 5'3" frame. When I reached 169 ½ lbs. I knew it was time to do something about it. That is when I went to Healthy Inspirations. The staff were so nice and promised me I would lose 10 pounds a month if I followed the plan and came in at least three times a week. Everything was so easy and I felt like family and they made me feel at home. Using their plan faithfully and the circuit and things I've learned at Healthy Inspirations has helped me stay in control.

Learning tips like having ready to eat foods in the refrigerator at all times has kept me from cheating. I've learned how to liven up dishes with spices instead of fat.

I was so impressed with Healthy Inspirations that I joined and I do not regret it at all. They have been supportive and encouraging each time I go. I have reached my goal and gone beyond. I'm now a vibrant person and exercise is a part of my daily life. I try not to go a day without it. I now have a boost of energy and I enjoy walking trails and bike riding with my children and grandchildren. What's really stuck with me the most is with every 5 pounds I lost, that's five pounds of sugar I'm not carrying around with me all day. Now, the bulging discs in my back do not hurt anymore, nor does the arthritis in my left side.

I've learned that by taking time for me and caring for myself, I'm better able to be there for others. Just look at me now! Thanks, Healthy Inspirations!

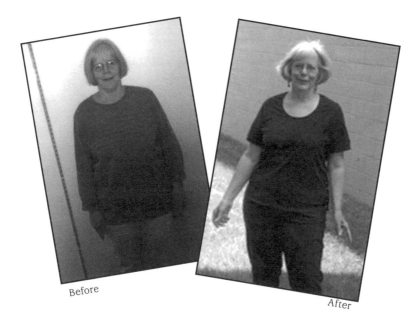

Before

After

Confession #26

May Guenin, Charlottesville, VA
22.2 lbs. lost

In high school it was easy. I shed excess pounds from childhood and paid attention to my clothes. Social attention, in the form of boy-friends, was my reward. I looked great and I have pictures to prove it! With the birth of my three children I gained but, again, I lost this weight. Whether this was youth or just my busy lifestyle, the effort, which I confess it took, did not seem extreme. When I worked there was always recognition for looking particularly nice, as well as for a job well done.

Trouble came in the form of an unhappy marriage. Pounds piled on and I had lots of difficulty taking them off. Yo-yo weight gain and loss followed. Even after I was divorced I found it hard to maintain a normal weight. There were years when I did well, but also years when my eating was out of control.

I went to my youngest son's high school graduation fat. I didn't want it to be that way. Four years later I went to his college graduation in the same dress. In addition to feeling bad about my weight, I felt bad about the fact that he had grown up; "Empty Nest Syndrome."

I've always liked food. My friends say I'm a good cook. Food became my solace. I was able to begin working part time from home, and I lost friendships I had enjoyed at work. Church and volunteering did not fill the void for me. Food did, unfortunately. I stopped buying clothes. I became more reclusive, more sedentary, more tired. At social events I would secretly count the number of overweight people. My doctor thought I was going through a "life phase adjustment." I no longer felt like myself.

I saw a nutritionist who prescribed a rather restricted 1200 calories a day diet. I lost some weight, but eating was boring. I regained my lost pounds. I was discouraged. A friend of mine had been going to Healthy Inspirations and lost 18 pounds. In the same length of time I had lost 15 pounds and regained them. I wanted the success she had. On her referral, I got a free health evaluation and more information about the program. I signed up.

One month later I had lost 14 pounds. Two months later I had lost 22.2 pounds. I met 40% of my goal! Three times a week I go into the Center for coaching. Pam cooking spray and Splenda are my best friends. I buy meat and fruit and repackage it in portion-sized servings. Salad mixings are always in my refrigerator. I turn down alcohol, bread and dessert at social functions.

I feel good again. I have more energy and I have more hope. I feel in control of my eating. I have clothes I used to love tucked away for use when I lose more weight. I get them out and try them on.

My son is getting married in a few months and already I know I won't have to wear the dress I wore for high school and college graduation. My hope is to wear a dress I made before he was born and have saved all this time for "just in case."

What made the difference for me? I think it is the staff, who always have a smile, always have a plan, and who takes the time to talk to me about my goals three times a week. They fill me with excitement about my success. I think they really care. I couldn't do this alone.

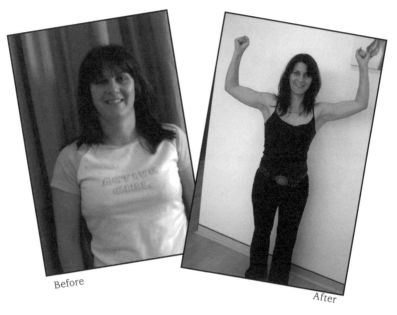

Before

After

Confession #27

Kathy Turner, Bunbury, Australia
24 lbs. lost

Somebody asked me the other day, "had I found the fountain of youth?" My reply was… "I found Healthy Inspirations."

I joined Healthy Inspirations in July 2005. My mission was to try to help repair my body of its ever increasing aches and pains, and decreasing the rise in body weight that was slowly rising with each passing year. I am a wife and mother of teenage children. My oldest was about to get her drivers license. This in itself was about to change many aspects within our lives. I was also twelve months away from turning 40.

Not being one to appreciate milestone birthdays, I was feeling rather weighted down and despondent as to what prospects the future would bring. Family play was an important part in my life. In return, I want to be there for my kids as they enter the sometimes rocky road into adulthood. I felt that I could not be at my best if I didn't feel and look my best. I needed to be able to have a positive outlook to cope with being a good parent of today's teenage kids. So with all this in mind, a friend came into work, sporting a new outfit and absolutely glowing with an inner self-confidence that I had never seen in this person before. That inner glow was certainly out there showing her new slimmer look. It was one of those moments where you would say, "I'll have what she's having!"

I made the phone call right then and there. I was confident that this was the Center for me. The moment I walked in I knew I had made the right choice. I was greeted with happy and friendly staff, willing to sit and listen to my individual needs and concerns. The Center was alive with women wanting the same as me. This was a big plus in that it was an all women's Center. Women of all ages and sizes, all with the same goals, all working hard to find that new healthier and fitter person within.

When the food program was explained, I knew that it was a realistic approach to eating. A sigh of relief that it was a lifestyle change that my whole family could embrace. I felt confident, too, that I had the knowledge and support to be able to implement this change without much sacrifice to their individual likes and dislikes. I was eager to learn the gym circuit. I had never been to a gym before, and never thought of myself becoming a gym bunny. But as the weeks progressed, I relished in my newfound strength. I was totally amazed after only a few weeks how my body was starting to mend its own aches and pains. As pounds were worked off, I looked forward to my visits. Whether it was a gram or a kilo, it was all a bonus and one step closer to my goal.

Before Healthy Inspirations, I dreaded that date in June and the big 4-0. But thanks to my friends at Healthy Inspirations and all of my hard work, turning forty will be exciting. I feel fantastic. I'm fit and healthy. I'm more confident and bursting with energy. I have achieved what I set out to do! I have lost 11 kilos (24 lbs.) in 8 months and lost 48 cm (18.9 inches) off of my body frame. I have gone from a size 14 to a size 10 in clothes. My daughter and I now share our clothes and the kids struggle to keep up. My family is very proud of my achievement and I thank them for their love and support, their encouragement and kindness, as they too have benefited from our new healthier eating and living plan.

This is only the beginning. It doesn't stop here. It only gets better. I am now equipped with the knowledge, help and support to sustain the new me. I feel calm, confidant and very reassured that my friends at Healthy Inspirations will be there for me; whether it's just for a word of encouragement to help me stay on track, or a welcome smile and a "glad to see you" on a day when you would rather go home than work on a circuit.

We all lead busy lives, so I have made exercise just part of what I do in a day. It is part of my everyday routine. I either walk or go to the gym. I try to do some form of exercise every day. It is now something I do without thinking of doing it or organizing it. It's amazing how much more I can manage to fit into my day. I think more clearly; I have more patience; I'm less stressed. Everyday is a good day. On bad days, well... they are few and far between.

So, have I found the fountain of youth at Healthy Inspirations? I think so. Not too many days go by without someone commenting on how fabulous I look. But my greatest gain and achievement is that I feel fantastic, it is that inner health and vitality, the whole new positive outlook, the feeling of calmness and rejuvenation, strength and well-being.

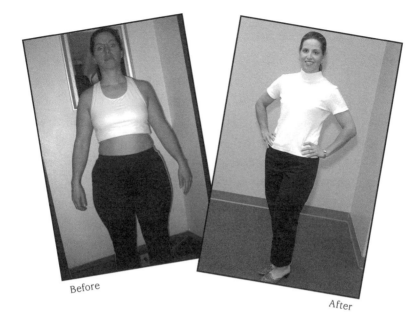

Before

After

Confession #29

Shelly Rutt, Lancaster, PA
20 lbs. lost

Last fall, I realized that after years of grueling workouts in the gym, I was not happy with the way my body looked or how I felt health-wise. I asked myself, "How could this be?" I ran 10 miles and had two days of free weights each week at the gym, plus I had a physically demanding job over the summer working for my father's landscaping business. I came to the conclusion that it was one thing that had pushed me into a size 14 and 166 lbs.- MY EATING! With a November 2004 sudden job loss that caused me to deal with depression, and working on three catastrophic natural disaster relief trips in 2005, I managed to gain 10lbs. in one year! I felt very out of control with regards to food. I began to ask myself some really tough questions about my uncontrollable cravings, emotional eating, and multiple weekly visits through the drive thru. I knew that my change would have to be deeper than a "diet." I participated in hypnotherapy to get to the root of my problem. It was helpful, but I still needed help on WHAT to eat to be healthy.

I met with the Director of Healthy Inspirations several times and finally committed to the program December 31, 2005. I started January 2nd. I loved the structure of the program and the food journaling. It was a complete overhaul of my typical eating regimen. I was extremely disciplined and determined to be successful in achieving a goal of 20 lbs. in 2 months. The program required me to forgo all my "emotional comfort foods" and within the first 3 weeks I really struggled with feelings of being emotionally "raw" or "exposed" since I absolutely could not hide behind my food any longer. Now, I knew I was onto something and really making life changes.

I supplement my nutrition and exercise program with vitamins, hormonal creams and the delicious Healthy Inspirations bars and hot cocoa. The Female Support hormonal cream had an amazing effect on my body! I have endometriosis and spent many of my 32 years in severe pain during my menstrual cycles. After using this natural hormone cream for just 6 weeks, I had no severe cramping, diarrhea, fevers, or days of lying in bed during my period! Amazing! Also, I was not nearly as "bloated" and continued to lose weight during the week of my periods.

I persevered for two months and met my goal of 20lbs. Additionally I lost 18 inches and now can wear all my size 8 clothes! The greatest feeling of achievement for me is when I stop and flex my muscles in the mirror and can FINALLY see all the years of working out since I took off much of the fat that was covering those beautiful muscles! As far as my eating, I am changed for life! I know how to eat now and I feel great eating organic, whole foods instead of the fast foods and chocolate candy bars I used to eat so regularly. However, I set aside a day that I eat a food that I enjoy that is not on the program. I do not feel like I am "missing out" or "sacrificing" anything since I have changed the things that I want and it feels SO good to wear all my favorite clothes again and clothes I never could wear before!

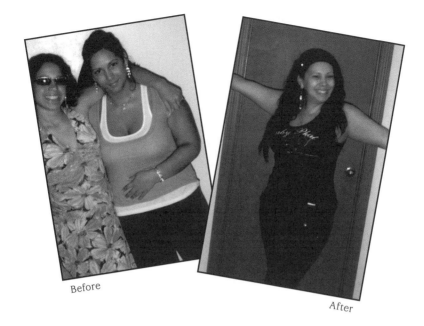

Before

After

Confession #30

Nicole Evans, Westerly, RI
22 lbs. lost

My name is Nicole and I'm 22. I love volunteering at the animal shelter, spending time with loved ones, music, fashion, and food! Within the past three months, I've been through incredible changes. I owe it to my sanctuary, Healthy Inspirations in Westerly!

Within four years, I gained 65 pounds, weighing more than ever. It came from slumps of laziness, depression, an unhealthy lifestyle of no exercise, an unhealthy diet and not caring, especially about what I was doing to my body, which was growing stretch marks and cellulite. Then came the worst insecurities and lowest self-esteem I've ever had. I couldn't fit into any of my clothes. I began to feel uncomfortable, not at ease with my appearance. I was utterly embarrassed. People would make comments about how pretty, but "heavy" I was. When I saw people, I was ashamed thinking they'd focus on my fattened status. My depression overcame me. All I did was snack and sleep. I was a miserable person. Finally in December, I needed a resolution I refused to give up on. I received a trial at Healthy Inspirations. I had to use my gift card to full advantage. It was time to make a change, to discipline myself to a healthy lifestyle.

I joined in January. I love the circuit! I'm committed to working out three times a week. The environment is welcoming and positive. The girls on staff have been absolutely warming and encouraging. They have a sincere, genuinely divine interest to help us in the most positive way. They have great substitutions for foods I need to cut back on. They make our Center enjoyable to go to, completing the process. I speak for many when I praise what great appreciation I have for them. All members are friendly and nonjudgmental, for in the end, we're all there for the same reason. I have recently referred my friend; our favorite thing is going to the "Girl Talk" meetings. It feels good to talk, listen, give and take advice, to relate to women who have struggled more than I wish to imagine. It's a place to build inner strength.

The results I've experienced include weight and inches lost. I'm swimming in pants I was bulging over! I weigh myself three times a month. So far I've lost 22 pounds. I have a better sense of well-being, energy, motivation and determination! My eating habits changed drastically! I watch what I eat. I allow myself one day out of the week to indulge in "naughty" foods normally avoided. My body feels healthier. I have a new sense of self-worth. I enjoy making constant plans and keeping busy. The most important result from working out is what a stress reliever it has become for me. I'm a very strong person, but I have a lot of anger inside. My biggest weakness is sweating the small stuff. When I work out, it's like I'm pushing all hate inside of me out and sucking all things I want in – happiness, peace of mind. I love working out because it makes my day brighter. It is my anger management.

My life has changed dramatically. I feel like that song, "moving on up", seeing only positives for the future. Physically, I have more stamina, endurance and strength. I'm more active and feel more alert. Emotionally, I'm grounded. I don't need anyone telling me who to be. I'm in control of my destiny. I've gained serenity. I feel beautiful both inside and out. I'm finally maturing, becoming the woman I need to be.

I'm not at my goal weight yet, but I'm not worried. I know my Healthy Inspirations team won't let me let myself down, even on low or bad vibe days. The most interesting fact is my success story doesn't compare to some in the program. I'm very fortunate and blessed considering many have more complicated, heart touching struggles and tasks of their own that they have conquered – sickness, illness, divorce and deaths of family members. They are an inspiration to me. Even though I'm not part of the actual team, I feel I could be or help give inspiration to other women. My life has gained ambition.

I feel wonderful! I'm glad I made the choice I love to share with the world – friends, family, patients, customers and strangers! I want everyone I know to make the change of direction to a happier, healthier life! Everyone deserves it and owes it to themselves! I have such a strong feeling of accomplishment already and extra confidence! It feels great when people tell me how great I look, when they notice and acknowledge my dedication and hard work! It lets me know all my effort was well worth it. Thanks to Healthy Inspirations, I'm inspired!

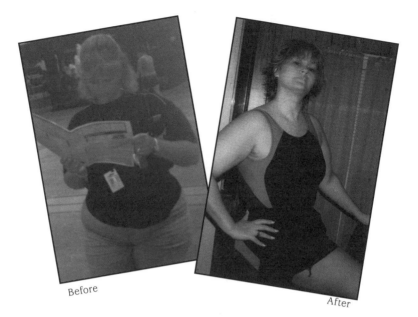

Before

After

Confession #31

Tammy Orndorff, Front Royal, VA
20 lbs. lost

Healthy Inspirations has been a godsend to me. Since I was twelve I
have been on some kind of self imposed "diet". My parents weren't
very supportive in my efforts; in fact my Dad's nickname for me
was "fatso." His whole family was overweight so I was genetically
impaired from the start. I had taken so many diet pills that I was
on the verge of Pulmonary Hypertension that almost landed me in
the hospital. I needed a plan that was centered around helping me
eat healthy and still lose weight without drugs, so after twenty-three
years and hundreds of failed attempts at losing weight, only to gain
it back and then some, I looked toward Healthy Inspirations for the
health and support I needed.

When I joined the program, I was amazed at the quantity of food
I could eat. I have never eaten that much throughout the day. The

thing that I appreciated the most was the support. There were days in the beginning when I would be on the verge of tears when I went to the Center, and with the help and support of the folks there I have been able to make it one more day.

I've been in the program now for five months and I have so much more energy, I sleep better and I have a better outlook on everything. My husband and kids say that I'm not as angry as I once was and my moodiness has leveled out. I've given away so many clothes that I have to buy more just to have something to wear, and it makes me feel great! I've lost a little over twenty pounds so far, which makes me so happy I feel like screaming it to the world! I look forward to getting on the scale now and seeing what tomorrow will bring.

I have never been one for exercise of any type, and it took me awhile to get into the groove of working out. Now I look forward to going to the gym, I'm eating things that I would have never tried before, cooked in ways that I would have never thought of cooking before.

Every aspect of my life has changed for the better and I am forever grateful to Healthy Inspirations for this, and can't wait to see what the future holds for me.

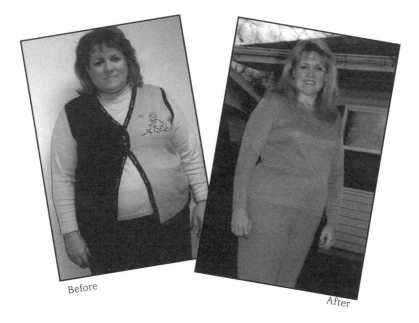

Before

After

Confession #32

Victoria Gillispie, Harrisonburg, VA
80+ lbs. lost

In January of 2005, I saw a friend that I hadn't seen in a while. She was half of her former self. I had been struggling with my weight, had tried all kinds of diets, programs, etc. and would always gain the weight back and more. I was so impressed with Dana that I asked her what she had done. She told me about Healthy Inspirations. I went to our local Healthy Inspirations and was horrified when the consultant told me that I was in the extremely obese category. I knew that I needed to do something because my Dad had open-heart surgery three years ago, and I could feel my heart beat in my ears when I bent over. The price quoted to me seemed high but I know that anything worth obtaining is going to cost you something.

What I like most about the program is the personable contact with the consultants. They are so encouraging and helpful, always willing to listen and answer any of my questions. I like having a plan to follow, and how easy the plan is to follow. I never liked exercise but I have gone faithfully to the Nautilus five times a week, and to weight in three times a week. I have enjoyed the monthly body comps, as I have been able to see pounds and inches melting away. With eating three meals and two snacks, I have never felt deprived.

I started out slow and kept at it, both writing everything down in my meal plan book and exercising. At the end of each week, I was rewarded with a nice weight loss. God has given me the strength and determination each day to go work out at the gym and to stick to my healthy plan. My husband has left an encouraging message on my voice mail everyday that I listen to as I drive from work to the gym.

My teenage daughters have also been a great support to me, helping to not cheat and telling me how great I look in my "new" clothes. It has been encouraging to have the diet consultants rejoice with me; sometimes they even have tears of joy in their eyes. Since last March, I have lost over eighty pounds and over sixty inches. I have gone from a size 3X to Lg/Ex, from size 26 to size 16.

My life has changed so much since then. I used to be very insecure and down on myself. I now feel very confident, pretty and very good about myself. I am a much happier person. I feel very strong now; I can bend over and tie my shoes and touch my toes; I can run and not get winded; I can race up steps and can still breathe when I get to the top. I have fulfilled one of my lifelong dreams. In October 2005, I ran and finished in a race that was over three miles long. I got to the finish line and cried tears of joy. I never thought I would ever be able to run again much less in a race.

I'm so thankful that God led me to Healthy Inspirations in March 2005, and that they were so kind and friendly on our first meeting. I am twenty pounds away from my goal, but I will get there, one step at a time, with my family and my Healthy Inspirations friends helping me all the way.

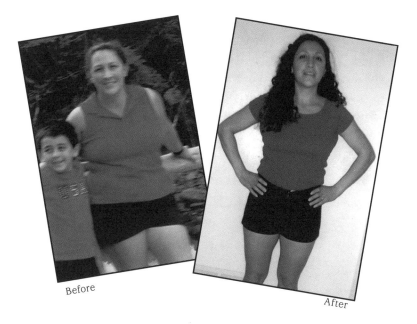

Before

After

Confession #33

Yvonne Merritt, Middletown, RI
40 lbs. lost

After having my third child, I felt tired all the time. I was overweight before I became pregnant and well, really overweight after. Although I was so very happy to have a healthy baby girl after my two boys, I was very unhappy with the way I looked and felt. My husband, a former Navy Seal, kept telling me that if I got back into shape, I would feel better.

Three months after having a c-section, I received a Healthy Inspirations ad in the mail with a lady's before and after picture. It explained that it was a healthy way to lose weight and a guarantee to lose three to five pounds a week! What a deal, it was just what I needed. I immediately called for an appointment.

I needed to lose at least forty pounds to get to a healthy weight that I would be happy with. I started at the end of August 2005 and the diet was working wonderfully. I immediately had more energy in just the few adjustments I made to my diet. Measuring and weighing is the ticket! We really do eat too much! I always forgot to eat fruit. The log really helped me to remember the good things that I was missing in my diet. I loved eating less [but] more frequently. The protein bars are so good; it was like cheating every time I had one. The exercise was fun, too! Once you got to know a few other women and got talking (as women do) you were done with your circuit. Thirty minutes is nothing. You know what they say, "Time flies when you're having fun."

Every time you reached a percentage goal you received a new gift, it was very motivating. When I reached my 20% goal I received a free t-shirt, 40% I received an aromatherapy treatment, then a facial and then a free Synergie treatment. These are all the things they offer in the Center to pamper yourself. They also have a room with a massage chair and soft music; it is a nice getaway place.

I lost an average of three to five pounds a week and once I saw results and started to fit into my old clothes, I was even more motivated to stick to the plan. I kept losing more weight, and the more people commented about my weight, the better I felt about myself. One of my friends commented that I looked twenty years younger. Also when I would go out to the grocery store with just the baby, everyone thought that she was my first baby. When I told them she was my third and my boys were eight and five they were shocked. I now have the energy to run along with the baby while my boys ride their bikes. We all love the time and togetherness we share. I am also able to take six-mile walks with my husband and run with him without complaining.

I feel so energized and happy. I am at my pre-babies weight and look much younger. When we went on a winter break it was hard for people to believe that I had an infant. I received so many compliments. It was fun!

My compliments to the program and the great support from the staff at Healthy Inspirations. I love the program and would recommend it to anyone.

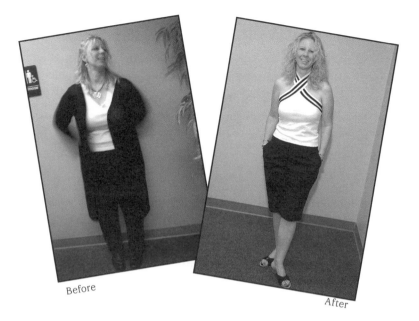

Before

After

Confession #35

Lisa Leeman, Lancaster, PA
40 lbs. lost

I am 39 years old and the Big 4-0 is quickly closing in. Age itself doesn't bother me, but I have definitely not been kind to my body during my 30's. My metabolism is slow despite a normal thyroid. Doctors told me I would have to monitor my weight and I believed deprivation was the answer, eat less and exercise more. I tried every diet fad and battled bulimia since an adolescent. Unfortunately, health has been another factor as I have had 9 operations in the last 7 years. Continuously I would lose weight only to regain more due to diet or health related issues. Eventually, I tipped the scale at 190 pounds. I needed help.

I spoke to a woman who told me about Healthy Inspirations. After my tour I was inspired! The program completely fit my ideals. Immediately I learned how to increase my metabolism. I thought they were crazy having me eat 5 times a day! I was never hungry. I found

I needed the accountability of writing down everything I ate. My journal helped me realize that I snack in the afternoon and eat when I am bored or lonely. This has helped me control my bulimia. Then it was enlightening to learn what a true portion size was. I found this to be an issue at home and in restaurants where portions were triple a true serving size. I ate well-balanced meals from each food group, and although I was skeptical, the supplements were not only filling, but also delicious and they satisfied my craving to eat something "bad."

I learned how to prepare my food and was surprised to learn that foods I once thought were good for me should actually be eaten in limited quantities. In addition to my diet change, I loved the exercise. Thirty minutes three times a week was so easy! I began to develop muscle and lose fat. It was working! Each week, stepping on that scale encouraged me for the next. The staff were always helpful and encouraging, mostly because they had participated in and benefited themselves from Healthy Inspirations. They understood and cared, so they empathized with my struggles and celebrated my successes.

The educational process had only begun. I learned the role stress plays in weight issues and was offered the use of a massage chair and sauna; both feel wonderful and rejuvenate body and mind. I learned the impact of hormones on total body wellness. This was essential information considering I had a hysterectomy at age 36. I now use their hormonal creams and am free from menopause symptoms. In 7 Synergie treatments, I lost 9 inches. I am amazed at the breakdown of fat deposits in my derriere and thighs. Healthy Inspirations continues to offer services and provide knowledge that inspires me to be my best.

There have been so many changes in my life aside from the obvious 40 pounds lost. More importantly than looking better, I feel better. I am healthier, happier and more self-confident. I am more active with my girls and more productive. I am a stay-at-home mom, but if I ever were to get a job, I would love to work at Healthy Inspirations and inspire others, as I have been inspired.

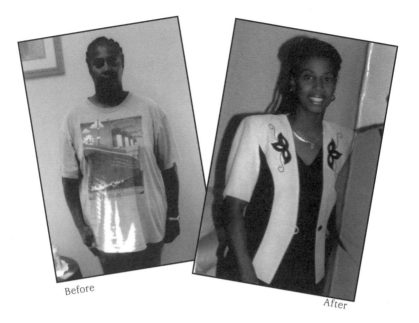

Before

After

Confession #36

Shirley Jones, Forest, VA
47.5 lbs. lost

OK, let's be honest. I'm a woman and I'm vain. I had lots of real reasons for finally taking the plunge and joining Healthy Inspirations. My blood pressure was up, my cholesterol was up and my body was not in the best shape. I was a big girl. Even as the scaled shouted a weight of 197 pounds, I believed I still looked good. Maybe that was because I have been bigger. At my heaviest, I weighed 235. I didn't want to admit it but I was fat. In fact, I was obese.

Probably not until I heard my own daughter imply that a certain size meant fat did a light bulb go on. While shopping with her in Atlanta, she became upset because she could not find the skirt she wanted. She wears a size 6. She commented that all they have are fat sizes when in actuality they had a size 12. The realization that my daughter thought that anyone size 12 and over was fat really struck a nerve.

I want to live and I want to be able to enjoy every aspect of my life. My daughter and I went to Hawaii last summer and I never once put on a bathing suit and got in the ocean because I was too ashamed of my body. When I came to Healthy Inspirations it was to get healthy, both physically and emotionally. I did not want to face another liquid diet. I wanted to eat regular food and see steady progress. That is what I discovered at Healthy Inspirations.

A student at school called me skinny the other day. Sometimes strangers are kinder to you. Of course, there are family and friends who are negative and try to discourage my decision to lose weight. I'm ok with that because I have never loved myself more than I do at this particular time in my life. I am a 55-year-old single mom. I have two adult children who are doing well. Now it is time for me. My birthday is April 1 and I plan to celebrate by participating in the 5K walk/run for cancer in Atlanta along with my youngest daughter. I couldn't have done this without the Healthy Inspirations program.

Healthy Inspirations has given me the confidence that I needed to lose the weight. Never once have I felt hungry or deprived of any foods. This is a diet for life. I am so proud of myself. I thank Healthy Inspirations and the staff here in Lynchburg. They were wonderful.

The physical weight loss is so exciting but I feel as if I have lost the same amount of emotional baggage. I have not been comfortable with how I have looked for a long time. I have always liked myself for my ability to deal with those things life has dealt me, but one look at my body would have told the true story. Healthy Inspirations has made me the person that I knew I was.

I would recommend this program and its staff to anyone who is serious about weight loss. I did it. Again, thank you Healthy Inspirations. I feel as if you saved my life. 56 won't be so bad after all.

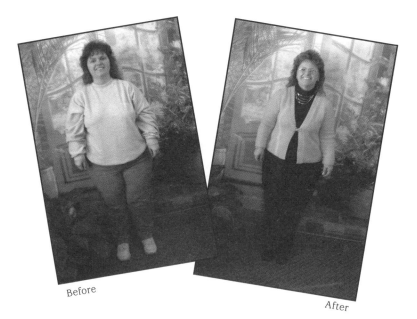

Before

After

Confession #37

Mildred Gehrke, Cottage Grove, MN
30 lbs. lost

I have been overweight for the last ten years. During this time, I have been complaining about my weight to my family, but I have done nothing about it. I had no willpower or ambition. The last year or so I had become depressed and stressed out. My oldest daughter heard an advertisement on the radio for Healthy Inspirations, and found that a facility was in our neighborhood. Without my knowledge, she contacted the facility and set up a consultation for me. On Christmas morning, as she was giving me my present, she asked me to keep an open mind and that she only wanted me to be happy with myself. I hesitated at first, but said ok. My present was a gift certificate for the first month at the facility. She told me that I had an appointment the next day for a consultation. I really didn't know what to say, except thank you. I wanted to keep the open mind that she asked of me, so I did. The next day we went to my consultation.

We were greeted with warm smiles. They were so happy to meet us, as they knew what my daughter had planned for me. They thought it was a wonderful gift. I sat there and listened to every word they had to say. I learned so much about myself that I didn't know. The person giving the consultation, the new knowledge and my daughter really inspired me to join. I knew that I could lose the weight so I started the next day.

What I like most is all the support that I receive. Not just the support from home, but the support from the staff at the facility. Every time I check in, I feel the support and warmth. This makes me want to work even harder, just to make them more proud of me. If I am having a week that the weight is coming off slowly, they educate me as to why. This pulls my willpower up another notch. The staff always takes the time to answer my questions. They share creative ways on how to prepare my food. This really helps me stay on plan, as I am a finicky eater. I also like the fact that the plan is grocery store food, and not diet food.

I have been on the program for less than three months, and have already lost 30 pounds. I have so much energy and willpower. I feel really good. The depression and stress are gone, and I feel like I have so much to look forward to. People at home, work, and the facility are all telling me how good I am looking. This helps me want to stay on plan, and work harder. While I still have 45 pounds to lose to make goal, I know that I can reach it, because of how good I feel today and the wonderful support that I have.

My life has turned around so much in the last three months. While I am no longer depressed or stressed out, I have gained so much energy and willpower. I enjoy so many things now, including my family. As I am still trying to obtain my goal, I do see a light at the end of the tunnel. I can't wait for all of the family activities to start in the spring and summer. We are all going to have so much fun, and I owe it all to my daughter and the staff at Healthy Inspirations.

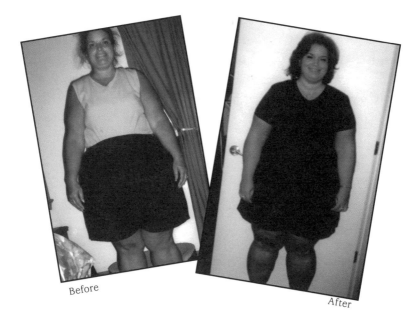

Before

After

Confession #38

Nancy Eagle, Charlottesville, VA
41.4 lbs. lost

I walked in the door of Healthy Inspirations on September 27, 2005. Little did I know how much opening that door would change my life. I had tried every diet know to "woman" on the market and was seriously considering gastric bypass. When I read about Healthy Inspirations I knew enough about nutrition to know that it all made sense. My only problem in the past was putting what I thought I knew into a plan that made sense…I was at my heaviest weight ever on that day, 282.6 pounds, and I knew that I could not hit the 300 mark. So, I signed up that day and today, April 24, 2006, I am 41.4 pounds lighter. I know that it is slow but I also know that I have changed my lifestyle forever and I will never be that heavy again.

Also, I was diagnosed with psoriatic arthritis in 1991 and that is a debilitating disease. I have to take two injections per week of Enbrel and two Indomethacin pain pills per day just to be able to walk. Since losing weight I still take the injections but there are days when I only have to take one pain pill and I don't have the joint aches that I did before. I am certain that all of this is because of my diet and exercise.

The thing that I like most about the program is the love and support that is given by the staff as well as my new "family" at Healthy Inspirations. I look forward to going to workout with all of my friends. We laugh a lot, compare stories, and since we are trying to achieve the same goals we feel comfortable with each other. We never feel like we have to be dressed up to go to a fashion show the way you are made to feel in other gyms, etc. Nobody cares if you have just rolled out of bed with no makeup on or hair done; I know this because that is me on Saturday mornings.

I have two grown children. My daughter is 25 and my son is 18. They have known me to be heavy all of their life. When they say things like, "Mom, it looks like someone took a needle and deflated your butt" or "Geez Mom, your legs are getting really skinny" that is enough to make you think, "WOW, it really is working". When your children are that proud of you there is no way that you can go back to the way you were.

The bottom line is that Healthy Inspirations has changed my life. I had never exercised before in my life on a regular basis. I now go 3-4 times per week and love it. I no longer eat any junk foods; as a matter of fact I don't even crave them anymore. I have more energy than I thought that I could ever have and I love myself more today than yesterday.

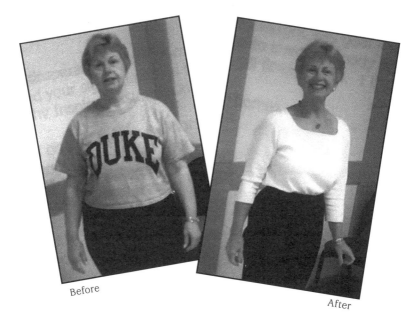

Before

After

Confession #39

Susan Thomas, Camp Hill, PA
23.8 lbs. lost

I felt desperate and out of control after gaining 30 pounds in three years. Even though I passed your sign numerous times, one day when I was stopped in traffic in front of Healthy Inspirations...I decided enough was enough!!!

Being one of the top realtors in the greater Harrisburg area, I am presented with daily challenges of an on-the-run, high-stress life-style. Feeling badly about my health, and myself, I was determined to find a plan that worked for me. Initially, I have to admit that I was a bit skeptical, however I soon learned, and was pleasantly surprised with how easy it was to adapt the Healthy Inspirations program into my extremely hectic schedule. What I like best about the Healthy Inspirations food plan is that it is well-balanced, nutritious, easy-to-follow... and, most importantly, they teach you WHAT food to eat and WHEN to eat them. My husband even had benefited from my joining Healthy Inspirations…he's lost 20 pounds, and we both have adopted a much more positive, active lifestyle.

Healthy Inspirations provides you with all the accountability, support and tools you need to succeed. You will lose weight because the program teaches you how to eat healthy grocery store foods, incorporate simple exercise into your life, and provide you with weekly relaxation treatments to control stress and overeating. All of this is done in a friendly, comfortable environment where you are given one-on-one attention and coaching, as well as the support and motivation you need to succeed.

I met my weight loss goal in July 2005. Not only have I maintained that goal, but I continue to lower my body fat percentage, increase my lean muscle mass and improve my overall fitness level. I look great and feel great!!!

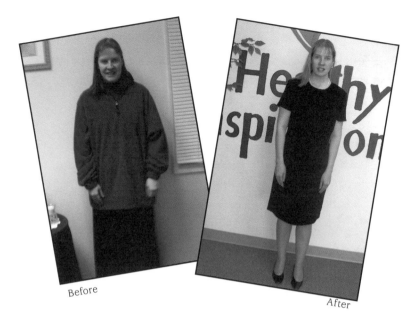

Before

After

Confession #40

Leigh Bruffy, Forest, VA
30 lbs. lost

Initially, I chose Healthy Inspirations for weight loss because a friend of mine had been there and she looked so dramatically different. I had wanted to lose some unwanted pounds for some time but I could never seem to find a "diet" that worked for me. I was not interested in "fad diets" because they only seem to work for a short while and then the pounds come back, usually doubled. Now that I had become a mother, it was increasingly important to me to get myself fit and learn how to eat right and stop the bad habits I had grown used to. I was giving my daughter a healthy lifestyle and I needed one too. That's when I decided to call Healthy Inspirations and make an appointment. It is one of the best decisions I ever made. The counselors are all helpful, friendly and knowledgeable and give all the encouragement you need to stay on plan. Healthy Inspirations truly cares about their client's health and well-being.

I went to Healthy Inspirations not knowing what to expect and wondering what they could offer that no one else could, I soon found out. Healthy Inspirations offers a unique approach to weight loss in that it is looked at as a lifestyle change. At Healthy Inspirations, you learn how to eat healthy and stay healthy with a balance of diet and exercise. The counselors teach you what you need to know about food, calories and healthy eating so that you can keep the weight off after reaching your goal. There is also a beneficial exercise program that keeps you toned and in shape while you are losing weight. Therefore, the results you achieve with the diet plan and exercise reflect a complete healthy image. Learning how to eat properly and keep my weight at my desired goal is what I like most about Healthy Inspirations.

Following the Healthy Inspirations plan, I have lost 30 pounds and I feel so much better. I was not overweight when I went to Healthy Inspirations. I had weight that I wanted to lose, but more than that I wanted to be healthy and stay healthy. With Healthy Inspirations, the weight comes off gradually which I understand is the best way to lose weight. I decided I was too young to be out of shape and have poor eating habits. The desire to set a good example for my daughter made the decision to enter the doors at Healthy Inspirations a snap.

Thanks to Healthy Inspirations, I have not only lost weight, but I feel so much better. I have much more energy, I am not tired all the time (due to improper nutrition), and my skin is no longer extremely dry because I know to keep myself properly hydrated. I now know that I can have chocolate once in a while, eat a slice of my daughter's birthday cake or let my husband take me out to eat for our anniversary and still maintain my weight. I am learning how to adjust my diet to allow for these special occasions. I was told by one of the counselors at the center, "you need to eat healthy 80% of the time and bad 20% of the time and not vice versa." I have found that approach to be most helpful to me. I would highly recommend this program. Healthy Inspirations has definitely changed my life for the better, in fact, when my weight loss is completed, the only thing big about me will be my smile!

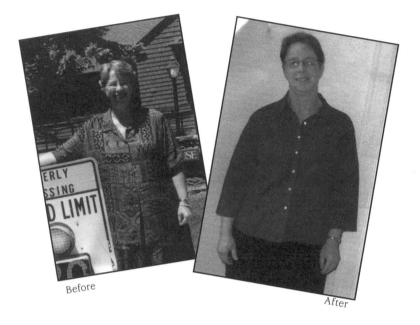

Before

After

Confession #41

Pamela Mott, Middletown, RI
20 lbs. lost

Going to any new place in life requires new tools, new information – if we are accustomed to the desert, the wintry northeast will require cold weather gear. Going through weight loss is no different. If we do not acquire and learn to use new tools along the way, no real progress will be made. I joined Healthy Inspirations to acquire and learn to use new tools. The old ones weren't working!

As I approach fifty, I want to be as healthy as I can be to do the work I love with as much energy as I can. I clearly needed new information and inspiration. Part of my journey is physical. At 70 pounds overweight, my health could be in jeopardy – I already knew the strain on my knees and a lower energy level. But part of my journey is spiritual – being willing to look at my consumption – my over consumption – in a world where many go hungry. I knew I had to use the tools at my disposal for myself and for a deeper connection to others.

Healthy Inspirations has provided a regular place to go for exercise and support. The women who work there have been caring and approachable. Sometimes that support has been humorous – I'll never forget Ruth saying, "You ate bacon! Ick, how can you eat that? It's so full of fat and salt!" I'll never be able to eat bacon in peace again! And that's a good thing! This relaxed environment of support has assisted my 20 pound weight loss in the past three months. I have about 50 pounds more to go but I feel as though I am learning new tools to get there. I realize you can't tell much from the "before and after" pictures – the weight loss shows mainly around my face; suffice it to say that I didn't keep many pictures before, and the picture taken at the Center was unavailable. I can no longer wear the blue outfit in the before picture because it is too big!

Healthy Inspirations promises that if you are 100% compliant with the program, you will lose 10 pounds a month. I wish I could say I was 100% compliant; I'm not. My life doesn't always allow for that. But I am learning simply to go back to the food plan as a way of life after an event or travel has derailed me. Learning to return to a healthy, intentional way of eating is important for the rest of my life, more important than the speedy weight loss. My thinking has changed in important ways. I finally realized that a burger and fries is not a treat. I would much rather have fish with heaps of fresh vegetables. My previous mindset would tell me that I could treat myself by having a burger and fries. Now I ask the question consciously: why do I think that this is the treat?

The women I have met at Healthy Inspirations are all on the same journey, all struggling with similar things. Everyone claps and cheers when a magnet is moved from 20% to 40%. We exchange stories of our lives as we work out, as well as healthy snack and meal ideas. New information, new tools, new friends…new inspiration!

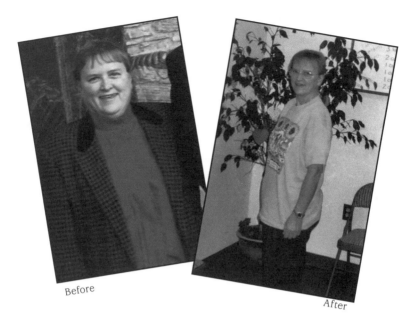

Before

After

Confession #43

Kathleen Wilson, Winchester, VA
65 lbs. lost

It was February 2004. I was still dealing with the loss of my eighty-year-old mother in April 2003. I had watched her struggle with many health problems including arthritis, high blood pressure, high cholesterol, and high triglycerides that I knew could have at least been minimized with weight loss.

I had struggled with my weight since I was a teenager. When I was about thirty-five I joined a weight loss program at the hospital where I worked and successfully lost about forty pounds and kept it off for about four years. I even became one of the speakers in the program to inspire other to lose. Then I changed jobs and got married and "little by little" the weight came back. I wasn't too concerned because I knew how to take it off, but somehow with age my metabolism had changed and the things that used to work didn't anymore! Suddenly, I was weighing more than I ever had in my entire life, two hundred fifteen pounds! My size eighteen jeans were too tight and I had to buy a size twenty! I was also struggling with high blood pressure, high cholesterol, high triglycerides and taking three different medications for it! I could only walk a short distance and felt winded. After attending my nephew's wedding in December of 2003, I looked at the pictures of myself and didn't like what I saw!

About that time I received an ad in the mail for Healthy Inspirations. What I liked about it was it guaranteed a one to two pound weight loss per week. I knew from past experience that this was the correct way to lose weight and decided to give it a try. I found the staff to be friendly and extremely helpful. The fact that all of them either were on the program or had been through it was encouraging to me. I also loved the massage chair as a great way to relieve stress! I continued on the program and by November of 2004 I'd reached my goal and lost sixty-five pounds and forty-eight inches! I gave away my size twenty jeans and now wear a size twelve, but more importantly I was able to reduce my blood pressure medication to half a tablet a day and I have more energy that I had when I was a teenager! I now do two miles on the treadmill and the circuit workout three times a week.

Thank you Healthy Inspirations! You have changed me for life!

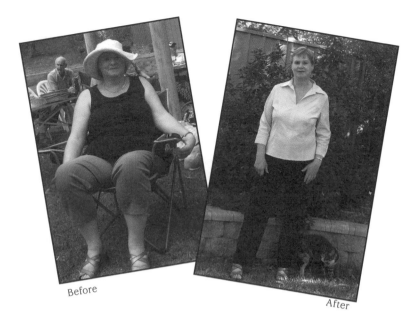

Before

After

Confession #44

Lesley Reilly, Blackwood, Australia
31.5 lbs. lost

It was my nephew's wedding in November that was the motivation for me joining Healthy Inspirations. I knew that there would be family photos taken and I knew that I didn't want to look like I did anymore.

So I started my journey in August 2005 after putting it off for a couple of months. I had seen the adverts for Healthy Inspirations soon after it opened but it took a while for me to realize that this could be the way to lose all the excess weight I had put on over the last few years.

I have thoroughly enjoyed my visits to Healthy Inspirations. The girls are very supportive and nothing is too much trouble. Not being one for exercise I struggled at first, but as I got fitter it became easier and now I look forward to my exercise sessions. Besides there is always a great bunch of ladies to exercise with as well as heaps of encouragement from the girls at the centre so how could you not enjoy it!

I've now reached 80% of my goal and have lost 14.3 kilos (31.5 lbs.) and 47.5 cm. (18.7 in.). I feel great and have so much more energy. An added bonus is my cholesterol levels have dropped and that has made my doctor very happy. There are times when I have lapsed (it took 3.5 months for me to move from 60% to 80%) but it is always easy to get back on the program. Just remember don't eat anything you wouldn't write in your journal!

My husband loves my new figure and it felt really good when people at work started noticing my new shape. I'm looking forward to reaching my goal and then maybe I'll set another one! So a big thank you to all at Healthy Inspirations – you are wonderful.

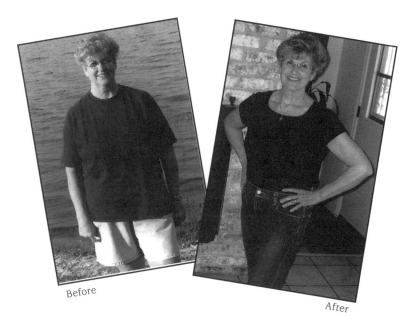

Before

After

Confession #45

Violet Smeltzer, York, PA
40 lbs. lost

Are you discouraged and feel you will never be able to look and feel the way you would like to? Please read my story and know your circumstance can change!

2005 was the beginning of a total life change for me and my family. I was sixty years old – having great difficulty walking and severe pain in my feet, knees and hands. I was looking at possible knee replacement in the near future. My cholesterol was not good and my blood pressure was high. The week of Memorial Day weekend, I was at one of my lowest points of feeling I would never succeed at losing weight. My husband wanted me to go with him to an open house at the fitness center he attended. I gave in and went. Healthy Inspirations was located at this center. He suggested I talk to them. I was greeted by a young lady who seemed to understand the way I was feeling.

She had lost over fifty pounds and looked terrific. It was great to talk to someone who had been where I was and told me I, too, could succeed. . .I was so excited! I really felt this might be the answer to a problem I had been dealing with for some forty years. I went for three days and decided to join.

I'm not going to tell you every day was a picnic, but even when I wasn't losing as fast as I wanted to, by the time I finished talking to the counselors and completed my exercise for the day, I was lifted up again. One of the most positive aspects of the program is the one-on-one counseling you have each time you go to the center. The counselors really listened to me and how I was feeling. They helped me believe in myself and not give up. They were always providing new recipes, which helped me to have a variety of things to eat. If I had a gain, I never felt like they put me down in any way, but they tried to get to the source of what I was dealing with that caused me to eat more. In this way, I was learning not to depend on food to be my comfort.

I reached my goal within five months time and have been able to lose ten pounds below my goal and feel great! My cholesterol is at normal levels and my blood pressure is under control. My knees and feet are feeling so much better without that extra forty pounds to carry around. I am now within five pounds of what I weighed when I was married forty years ago!

Everyone has encouraged me so much. It is so much fun to go shopping and buy smaller sizes. I praise God for leading me to Healthy Inspirations and changing my life forever. I would like to encourage YOU to know your life too can change. Check out the program and begin to believe in yourself again. Life is too precious to give up.

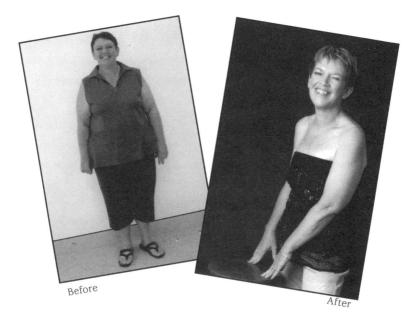

Before

After

Confession #46

Judy Taylor, Tamworth, Australia
77 lbs. lost

Everyone has a "thorn" in their side. Mine was being overweight. I had lost weight many times and I knew just about everything there was to know about food, exercise, diets and everything associated with it. I knew losing weight was about more than what I ate and how much I moved. Healthy Inspirations came along at the right time and a friend of mine just happened to be one of the consultants. She gave my husband her card, in case I was interested. No reason not to be – I was going through one of those "I'm fed up" stages and was willing to give anything a go. When the program was explained to me, everything fell in to place. The eating plan was easy to follow, needed no special food and, from what I knew about diets, was well balanced, including all the food groups. The exercise plan made sense too, combining aerobic exercise and the promotion of muscle development. Best of all, the relaxation component was something no other program I'd been on had thought of. In my stressful job, the thought of sitting for 20 minutes a week and doing nothing was heaven. Even the price and the method of payment were just right for me. I was sold!

I discussed my goals with my consultant. Having achieved thin-ness before, I knew what was in store for me. This time however, I was a bit more realistic. My consultant listened to me and respected the things I told her, giving sound advice based on these things. I not only wanted to lose weight, I wanted a whole new lifestyle; one which took into account my physical and mental well-being. The Healthy Inspirations program offered all of this. We set a goal weight and decided then and there the times for my centre visits and even when I would use the relaxation chair for the first time. I appreciated the gentle encouragement and support as I started on this new road and was determined to give it my heart and soul. "Fifty and fabulous" was my motto and my goal.

I feel great – eating healthy and exercising regularly – it's a new life-style I am keen to maintain. There is even a plan for when your goal weight is reached. This was a worrying time for me as I'd lost a lot of weight before, only to put it back on in a short period of time. I still occasionally fall off the "wagon" but at least I have a "wagon" to get back on to and lots of friends to help me.

Everything about my life has changed. I can't think of one area that has stayed the same. There's the obvious changes: eating healthier meals, exercising regularly, fitting into that size 12, being able to wear swimmers again, more energy, etc, etc. The biggest change I've noticed is that I now have the confidence to look after (take care of) myself. My health is now my priority because without it, I won't be around to enjoy anything else. The most dramatic changes that are still taking place are in the thoughts that go on inside my head. It's been a struggle to stop thinking like a fat person. I am getting used to seeing myself in the mirror – my reflection used to surprise me in the early days. If I eat too much, it's not so much of a struggle to get back to eating to plan. That's where the centre and the consultants come in handy. They are always so complimentary and willing to share in your highs and lows. I am starting to accept the fact that I am OK if I eat something I shouldn't and that if I put on a kilo, it only takes a return to plan and a bit of exercise to get it off. It's a lifetime venture, changing that hopeless mindset.

The best change I've noticed is that I now have become an inspiration for other people. I think everyone would like to leave this world knowing they've made a difference. Healthy Inspirations has allowed me to do that. By using my story and photos, people I know and don't know have been motivated to start making the same changes as I have. It is so uplifting to have people come up to me and say: "I'm here (at the centre) because of you" or "Your photo in the paper has inspired me to start losing weight". Not to mention the fact that it keeps me on track, knowing I'm a role model for others and that they are watching me and taking their lead from me. If you're contemplating hopping on the merry go round again, try Healthy Inspirations. Give it everything you've got for as long as it takes – it's worth it and it works.

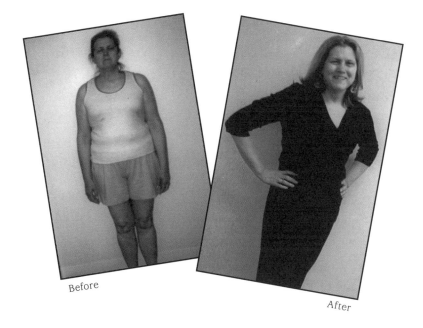

Before

After

Confession #47

Joanne Breslin, Cranston, RI
30+ lbs. lost

I kept telling myself I could get rid of those few extra pounds any time I wanted. Just eat less, exercise more. Time passed, those few pounds become many, and multiple abdominal surgeries took their toll. I kept telling myself I could take off those extra pounds whenever I wanted.

Health problems – some major, some minor – exacerbated the situation. I knew getting my weight down could help, but hey, the medication was working and besides, wasn't weight gain a possible side effect? Health problems can cause stress and stress can cause weight gain, right?

More problems, more stress, more medications, more weight…you get the picture.

The day I was diagnosed with non-alcoholic fatty liver disease (NAFLD) was devastating. Left untreated, it could lead to sclerosis of the liver. The disease was in its very early stages, though, and my doctor felt confident it could be reversed by weight loss. I joined Healthy Inspirations the next morning.

Emotionally, I was a wreck. The Healthy Inspirations program seemed to make good sense, though, and it did seem thorough: healthy diet, doable workout program, that amazing shiatsu chair to relieve stress. The counselors were knowledgeable, confident of the program, and excellent listeners. They realized my problems, fears and goals were unique, as everyone's are.

In the general scheme of things, I didn't have that much weight to lose: my goal was 30 pounds...and changing my lifestyle. Too much was at risk if I didn't.

Phase 1 (the quick-start part of the plan) went well. But the first real test came after I started Phase 2. I was very emotional at that first weigh-in. After such a short time, I absolutely loved this new way of eating! My husband, the cook, had promised to follow the plan to the letter. It took only days for us to know this was the way we wanted to eat for the rest of our lives. Food tastes so good prepared according to the guidelines. The variety and the quantity were perfect. The workout seemed almost too easy. But would the results be there?

They were. And I have never looked back. My (our) new lifestyle is absolutely amazing. I lost my 30 pounds, and set a new goal of 10 additional. The first 30 were for health...the next 10 are for me.

Was it easy? Surprisingly, yes. That's not to say things always went smoothly. I was lax in working out, especially at the beginning. But I got better and saw quick results. Most weeks my stress level was very high. Life happens, and it happened to throw me some nasty curves.

I reached my initial goal about a month ago and have had time to reflect how that has changed me. Very happily, my liver problems have diminished. I'm now working on reducing the amount of medication I have been taking for other health issues. That may not be possible, but at least I will know I am not sabotaging my health.

I feel great and look even better. My confidence is at an all-time high…so is my humility. I realize how lucky I am not only to have a wonderful husband and alert doctor, but an amazing program and caring staff at Healthy Inspirations.

Just a few days ago I ran into a friend I hadn't seen since just before I joined Healthy Inspirations. She raved about how wonderful I looked and asked for the particulars. When I told her the story, she said, "Joanne, you inspire me!" Thanks, Healthy Inspirations!

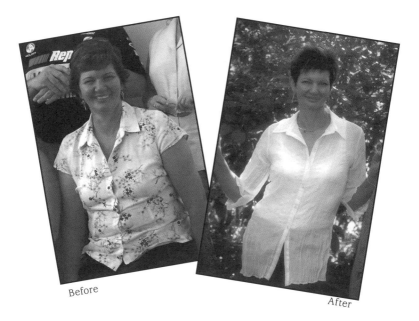

Before

After

Confession #48

Sandra Cosford, Kenmore, Australia
35.2 lbs. lost

It was back in March 2005 that I finally realized that I had to do
something about my weight. All the ladies in my family are large and
until then I had tried hard to avoid joining them but I was losing
the fight. I was out of control and getting steadily more depressed.
My husband had pointed out kindly that I would have to buy some
new clothes, as the stretched material and straining buttons were not
attractive. He even went out and bought me a whole set of very plain
clothes in size 16 as if to make the point that I was no longer young
and stylish. Then I had a family photo taken in the back yard and
that proved to be the call to action that I needed. The sight of my
pudgy face and the rolls around my middle forced me to make the
decision to get back in the driving seat and take control of my life
again.

I knew that latching on to fashionable diets and get-slim-quick routines was not going to work and I knew I needed help if I was to make real and lasting progress. I have strong self-discipline but I needed to have structure and support if I was going to success. I scanned the local papers and chanced upon an advertisement for Healthy Inspirations at Kenmore. So I called in for an appraisal. The friendly reception and the positive atmosphere quickly dispelled my apprehension and I decided to enroll. It was the balanced, life-style approach that appealed to me, not just watching what I eat but adjusting my routines, taking regular exercise and thinking about what I was doing. With their help I set realistic, achievable targets and started slowly on the path to a new life.

One year later, I have not only lost 16 kilos (35.2 lbs.), but I feel so much fitter and healthier. I eat well and don't have to stick to special diets or eat special food. I have given away all my size 16 clothes and replaced them with a whole wardrobe of size 12 and even size 10. I feel good about my appearance and my self-esteem has soared.

It's not just about losing weight; it's about changing the way you think about yourself and your lifestyle. To make a lasting change takes discipline and time but the rewards far outweigh the effort. For some people a size 10 outfit is something they take for granted; but for those of us who have a tendency to put on weight, a size 10 dress is a triumph, a kind of trophy, the result of a balanced program of diet and exercise. The team at Healthy Inspirations has been really wonderful. From being my support group they have become my friends. My visits to the gym are not so much a chore or an effort, but a pleasurable way of spending an hour two or three times a week.

Thanks to Healthy Inspirations, I am now back in charge of life, looking and feeling better that I have for 20 years. Talk to Healthy Inspirations, listen to the advice of their experts and follow their plan. Believe me, it really works!

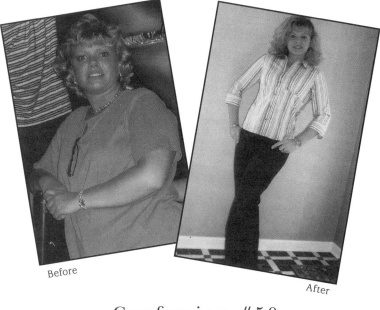

Before

After

Confession #50

Caryn Brown, Forest, VA
49 lbs. lost

Healthy Hope! Healthy Life! Healthy Inspirations!

Full figured, plus sized, large and lovely, no matter how delicately
I tried to label it, I was fat. Because I had tried and failed at other
plans (Weight Watchers, New Weight, South Beach, Atkins, to name
a few), I had lulled myself into a false acceptance of my oversized
figure. I thought that I was okay with my size until my mother mentioned that she had seen a relative who had great weight loss success
with Healthy Inspirations. And as my mother put it, "If she can do
it, you can too". That really touched a nerve with me. I felt a twinge
of desire to be different. Apparently I was not at all right with my
fatness after all. I was thirty-one years old, obese (size 18+) with high
blood pressure, no exercise tolerance, and I was eating my way to
diabetes and heart disease.

The Healthy Inspirations way gave me a glimmer of hope. What most impressed me about the program was the support and encouragement that was provided. Healthy Inspirations was unlike any weight loss plan that I had ever encountered. The friendly Lifestyle Consultants met with me three times a week and held my hand as I baby stepped my way through 49 pounds of excess weight. The structure, nutritional education, support and encouragement that were provided to me are the reasons for my success.

What is so amazing is that the Healthy Inspirations plan actually lives up to its claims! I followed the nutritional guidelines, exercised using the circuit, ate sinfully delicious protein snacks and lost an average of 2.5 pounds per week. The steady progress is motivation in itself. And more importantly, I was never hungry!

Everyone around me has watched me change. People frequently comment on how good I look (in my new size 8 jeans). My results have even motivated others to examine themselves, their lifestyles, and their desires. Three of my co-workers have enrolled at Healthy Inspirations and two others are contemplating their decision.

Currently I am in the Healthy Balance portion of my Healthy Inspirations plan. I have lost a total of 49 pounds and counting. I have gone from a size eighteen to an eight. My health is much improved. I no longer require medicine for high blood pressure, and my cholesterol is down. My energy level is through the roof! I can ride my bike, I can run, I can play with my son even after working as an RN in a busy operating room.

Thanks to Healthy Inspirations, my future is bright and filled with hope. I am winning the weight battle. I am revived and I am alive! What a blessing!

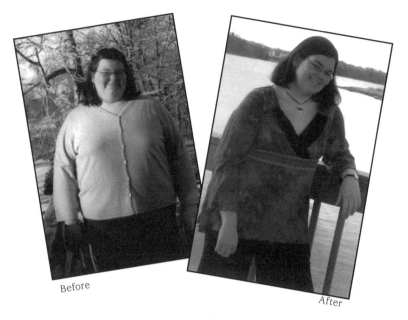

Before

After

Confession #51

Christine Daylor, Wakefield, RI
93 lbs. lost

Imagine having to live the rest of your life with an incurable disease. This is the reality that was facing me as I sat in my doctor's office last summer. I was there for my annual physical when I pointed out some dark, rough skin on the back of my neck to my pediatrician. After looking at it, she told me it was a warning sign for insulin resistance, and that if I didn't do something to correct it, I would become diabetic. This was a big concern considering both my grandfather and uncle have diabetes.

At 337 pounds, I was far from a healthy teenager. I was sixteen years old and having to live the rest of my life testing blood sugar twice a day was not what I wanted to do. I'd been extremely overweight throughout my childhood, but now it was life threatening. I needed to do something. I'd tried dieting on my own before, but nothing worked. My doctor recommended Healthy Inspirations to me, a diet and exercise center just for women. I went to a consultation meeting with my mom and signed up for a year of membership.

The first week was pretty rough having to deal with the thought of not eating all my favorite foods like chocolate, ice cream and pasta. I told myself I would never be able to do it. But the girls at the Center were supportive and encouraging, and I lost seven pounds in my first week. After that, I just kept myself motivated and told myself I was strong and could follow the program along with my schoolwork. I love the atmosphere of the Center. Everyone is always upbeat and friendly, and when you walk in, you're filled with energy. The circuit really helped me step up my exercise level, and after the first two weeks, I had more energy than in the last two years of my life. Probably my favorite part of the program is the specific eating plan the consultants picked out for me. They matched my needs as a borderline diabetic to a certain plan for me that has helped me lose weight safely and lower my insulin level. I know this because all the dark, rough skin on the back of my neck has gone pink and smooth.

I've been on the program for seven and a half months, and I'm now seventeen. I've lost ninety-three pounds and weigh 244. I feel great about myself and what I have accomplished. After participating in this program and succeeding, I know I can do anything I put my mind to. Relatives that I don't see for a month or two always say I look great, and my friends and even teachers at school are noticing I'm slimming down. I have the most self-esteem I've ever had. Mean comments in the hallway no longer bother me because I know that I'm working on getting my weight down. Junior prom is coming up in two and a half months, and I can't wait to go dress shopping because I've never worn a dress before in my life. But now I have the confidence and slimmer shape to feel good about myself and the way I look. I don't have to worry about living with diabetes, and I know that I'll live a long, healthy life. I never could have done it without Healthy Inspirations, the excellent program, and most of all, the encouragement and support from all the girls who work there.

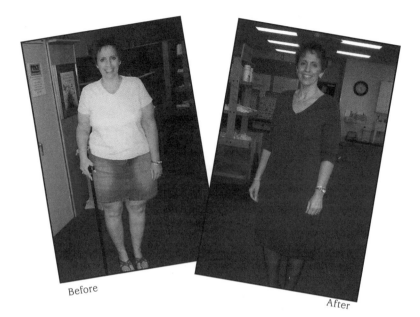

Before

After

Confession #52

Vina Landis, Germantown, PA
111 lbs. lost

I joined Healthy Inspiration as a Multiple Sclerosis (MS) patient looking for something to improve my quality of life through weight loss, muscle building and proper eating. Three times, I lost the use of my legs and was told that I would never walk again. Yet, I was able to recover. To do so, however, meant lots of physical therapy along with many medications, including heavy dosages of steroids. Unfortunately, the side effect was a large amount of weight gain.

When I began to walk again, I knew I had to get the rest of my body back into shape. Even though I could walk, I simply did not feel well physically or emotionally. I weighed 272 pounds and was ready for a change. I began to eat better and lost 62 pounds by cutting down on unhealthy foods. However, it was clear that I needed a much more focused, lifestyle changing program if I was to lose the amount of weight desired and build the muscle needed to combat my MS. That is when I joined Healthy Inspirations.

I had tried several programs before, but found this program targeted both weight loss and muscle gain using a realistic approach. What I liked most about it was that it seemed easy to follow. Unfortunately, one of my MS symptoms is cognitive difficulties. Therefore, I needed a program that was uncomplicated; otherwise I simply couldn't do it. The Healthy Inspirations program delivered. I was able to easily understand the eating changes I needed to make. There weren't difficult mathematical computations or recipes to follow. I knew I could do it and off I went.

After losing 20 pounds, I began the more physical part of the program and found my new best friend, Pilates. In the past, exercising was difficult because of the physical and cognitive issues affecting my ability to keep track of what exercise I was doing and counting repetitions. With Pilates, I was able to follow the routine. Soon, I was able to do the exercises alone and was a workout addict. So much so, that an article was written about me in our local Gazette newspaper explaining how I was combating MS with the Healthy Inspirations program.

I was so proud of what I had accomplished. By that point, I had lost 49 pounds, was eating right and was simply feeling better than I had in years. I was seeing and feeling muscles on my body that I had not remembered were there and was actually pointing out my new muscles to others. My life was truly transformed. I had more energy to accomplish my day-to-day tasks as well as begin a more active social life again. I was more confident and looked forward to clothes shopping once again. My relationships with others also improved, because of this newfound energy and self-confidence. My friends and family were certainly proud of me, and happy to see me in such good health. But, I was more proud of myself. I stuck with it and was able to do what I set out to do. Physically and emotionally, I was alive again. I told everyone I could about this program and continue to do so today at health fairs. I am often told how much people admire me for the transformation I have been able to make in my life and that I inspire them. I love to think that my success has lead and will continue to lead the success of others. To me, that is the cycle of true inspiration.

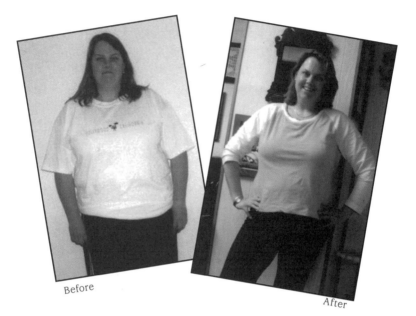

Before

After

Confession #53

Jennifer Kane, Middletown RI
70 lbs. lost

I am so inspired that I put it all in print – weight, measurements and my age! And all in a local newspaper for everyone to see!

I joined Healthy Inspirations in January 2004 with a weight of 260 pounds. I, like so many other people, have always had a weight problem. I was always heavy and year after year my weight crept up. In February 2002, I had my first child. After Rose-Ellen was born, I lost all but 10 pounds of my pregnancy gain. Then in August 2003

Emma arrived, and I kept another ten pounds. I was at a very unhealthy weight and wanted to do something about it.

A friend and I had decided to get serious about our health. We were each going to research some of the area weight loss options, and I walked into the Middletown Center. Healthy Inspirations had so much more to offer than anything else out there. I was very impressed and excited about weight loss and nutrition counseling in one place.

This was the first time in my life I was ever serious about a weight loss program. I had tried different exercise programs but had never been able to stick with anything. The circuit workout at Healthy Inspirations is so perfect – it changes every month and helps to keep things from getting monotonous. I started looking forward to working out. It was such a nice change from dreading the gym. Now, I am at a point where I feel so great after each workout.

Three weeks ago, I reached my goal. I have lost 70 pounds. It was such a great moment – adding my name to the 100% list. It has been such a wonderful experience, one that I have been able to share with friends and family. I have friends that have joined Healthy Inspirations after seeing how great I have done.

In January of this year, a local newspaper contacted Healthy Inspirations about doing a story. They wanted to follow three women for a year in their journey to good health. I was very nervous about being part of this story – but I went for it. The day we met with the reporter was scary! She asked for all the measurements and our weights. I don't know why this was a surprise to me. It was going to be a story about weight loss – of course they would need to know our weight. When the first article came out, I had a major anxiety attack. There we were – on the front page of the paper. I couldn't help but wonder – what have I done? Then I received some great phone calls. People that I hadn't spoken to in awhile called to support me. I received an amazing letter in the mail. This person thanked me for having the courage to put my story in the paper. She had been struggling with her weight and health for a while. After reading the article, she joined Healthy Inspirations. The letter made all the anxiety worthwhile.

There have been three articles so far. Now I look forward to seeing my picture and measurements in the paper. The inches and pounds go down, and the pictures are looking better.

Last week, I ran into a new member at the Center. Ten years ago we worked across the street from each other, but I haven't seen her in awhile. She told me she had seen the paper and that I had inspired her to join and get healthy. It really is a great thing. I'm getting healthy and helping out some other ladies at the same time.

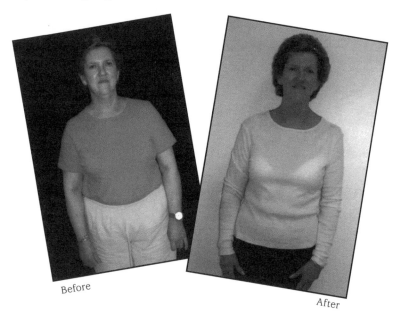

Before

After

Confession #54

Mary Louise Leake, Fishersville, VA
38.8 lbs. lost

Almost nine months ago I joined Healthy Inspirations. Rather ironic, the timing. In the time it takes to give birth, I too have begun a new and healthier life, to last forever.

In July 2005 I was miserable. My clothes were tight; suit skirts went unbuttoned under jackets, lovely size 10's were waiting in the closet while I stuffed myself into 16's. I refused to buy more "fat" clothes, so outfits were limited. I had a new sports car that I loved, but felt like I had been squeezed into the seat. My swollen, painful left knee was nearing the replacement stage and prevented aerobic classes. Looking in the mirror, I saw jowls in my face and large pads of fat on hips and thighs...my body was changing and this final weight gain was the cruelest of all.

I have battled my weight since childhood topping 317 pounds in my early 20s. I lost 182 pounds previously and kept it off for twenty-five years. In my late 40s, the numbers climbed to the 180 mark and I lost again to about 145. In 2005, my 57th year, I hit 178. In July I saw a TV ad for Healthy Inspirations. I checked it out and knew it was the program for me!

There is no one best thing about Healthy Inspirations. It is the ultimate lifestyle program for diet, exercise and relaxation. I never cheated. I didn't need to. Everything is under one roof, you are never hungry and never have cravings (thanks to the supplements!), you have individual counseling and support, the exercise is great and low-impact (my knee looks and feel great!), the weight loss (both pounds and inches) at age 57 with slower metabolism is phenomenal. The weight loss has never been easier, more satisfying or healthier. The visuals used in the program are both clever and motivating. Lavender ribbons cut to corresponding inches clipped to each journal are constant reminders and trophies of my hard work and accomplishment!

I am wearing size 8's and my size 10's (altered) that were waiting for me. I am now 9 pounds below my goal weight of 137.98, with a starting weight of 167.8! My lowest weight ever! My skin and nails have never been healthier due to the diet and the EFA's. I use the relaxation chair weekly and treat myself to a full body massage monthly. The results are truly amazing. My counselors asked me to be the "Poster Child" for the local Chamber of Commerce flyer for advertising Healthy Inspirations.

My life has changed dramatically these past 9 months. So many people have asked me how I have lost weight and how the pounds seemed to just disappear. I keep Healthy Inspirations information with me everywhere. I am proud to say that I have brought 7 new clients to my Center. I want other men and women to feel as fit and healthy as I feel. Healthy Inspirations has helped me become a healthy inspiration to others. How do I know this lifestyle is forever? I love the way I look and feel in my clothes. It is truly the first time in my entire life that when I look into the mirror, I see, feel and know I am thin. It is the first time ever that I am comfortable with how my body looks and feels. This is me, the last and best me!

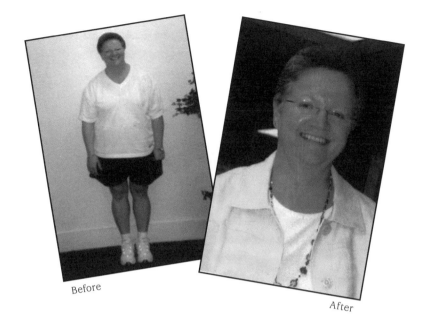

Before

After

Confession #55

Debbie Shelor, Charlottesville, VA
40 lbs. lost

According to Webster, healthy means "enjoying health and vigor of body, mind, or spirit," and inspiration is "the process of being mentally stimulated to do or feel something." For me, Healthy Inspirations has come to mean the process of being mentally stimulated to enjoy health and vigor of body, mind and spirit!

One year ago, I picked up a flyer, walked through a door, and set foot on a path to change my life. After years, even decades, of being overweight, the time and circumstances were finally right for me to do something about it. Several events brought me to this point... missing my high school reunion (twice) because I didn't want my old friends to see how overweight I had become, the shame I felt from making up excuses to avoid hikes and other physical activities because I didn't have the stamina to participate, seeing my doctor write "obesity counseling" on my chart during a routine physical, having to take medication for high cholesterol and high blood pressure, caring for my mother during major surgery to counteract her congestive heart failure, and the opening of the new Healthy Inspirations Center in my city.

In 1999, I had joined another popular weight loss program and lost 25 pounds. Without my even realizing it was happening, I gained all the weight back in less than two years, which left me feeling totally defeated and convinced that I would never be able to lose the weight and keep it off. All of that changed last April when I joined Healthy Inspirations. Right from the start of my first orientation session, the lifestyle consultants made me believe that I could lose the weight and keep it off. They convinced me that this program would work for me. They taught me that it's about so much more than losing weight...it's about getting healthy! And that's just what I've spent the past year doing.

Thanks to the healthy eating plan, reduced sodium intake, water-drinking regimen, regular exercise and relaxation, I am now 40 pounds lighter, a great deal stronger, physically and emotionally, and much healthier. My cholesterol has decreased dramatically and my blood pressure now stays within a healthy range – without medica-tion! The convenience of weighing in, exercising, and relaxing at one location was easy to fit into my busy schedule as an elementary school teacher. And the regular coaching and counseling has seen me through every rough spot and every milestone of success.

My accomplishments have been obvious to my family, friends and even acquaintances in a variety of ways. Going from a size 18+ to a size 10 in clothing has prompted comments like, "Wow, you look fabulous!" and "You look like an athlete" and "You look like you're 25 years old in that cute little skirt!" (an enormous compliment for a 45 year old woman). The first time my father saw me after I'd lost a noticeable amount of weight, he said, "Well, I didn't realize I still had a little girl in the family." But even more important than having people notice the change in my physical appearance has been the acknowledgement that I have changed as a person. Having a colleague say, "You just exude happiness and confidence these days," and hearing my best friend declare, "I've never seen you look so happy," just reinforced my own realization that I have accomplished something truly monumental. With the guidance of the Healthy Inspirations program and the love and encouragement of my lifestyle consultants, I really have been inspired to get healthy and stay that way.

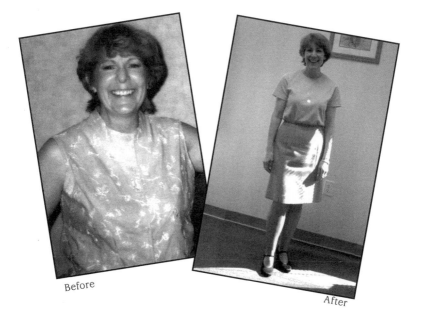

Before

After

Confession #56

Diane Bort, Forest, VA
25 lbs. lost

Dear Healthy Inspirations,

Thank you so much! You did what you guaranteed you could do: you helped me lose 20 pounds by the end of the year. I joined the program in mid-October and by December 31, I had lost the weight I had been trying to lose for the past 15 years.

In the past, I tried other exercise and diet programs. They were very well known and reputable programs. Some had me buy their food, which I did. EW! How long can you eat prepackaged foods before you go broke or get sick of their food? Some of them had me adding up points all day long. I would eat my entire points in junk food some days. What kind of plan was that? I also tried my own, trying to eat sensibly. Less calories in, more calories out. You know, decrease the amount of food I can eat and exercise more. I thought, "I'm a nurse, I can do this." Wrong again. I would always lose a few pounds at the beginning and then fall back into my old eating habits. Before six months were up, I would have gained all the weight back plus a couple more pounds. I always felt hungry.

At Healthy Inspirations, you taught me how to eat properly so that I don't feel hungry. You gave me one-on-one counseling several times a week to help me stay on plan. And you were always available by phone if I had any questions. You also gave me a place to come and exercise painlessly! And the massage chair became my new best friend. The chair helped me realize just how stressed I could get. My back and neck would be so tight. But by the end of the 30 minutes in the chair, I was relaxed and calm. My outlook on life would be so much better! I am still at my goal weight this March 21! And I have even lost a few more pounds!

I really like your program and recommend it to everyone who asks me how I lost the weight. I like the fact that I eat regular food that I buy at the grocery store. I eat healthy meals: meat, vegetables and fruit and healthy portions of starches. And I enjoy the supplement bars. The little bit of chocolate every day really helps me stay on the plan without feeling deprived.

I have learned a new healthy way of eating and I plan on sticking to it for the rest of my life. And I have some new friends, too! Thank you (to the Healthy Inspirations staff) for all your help and inspiration. You helped me to feel better about myself. My health has improved and my appearance, too!

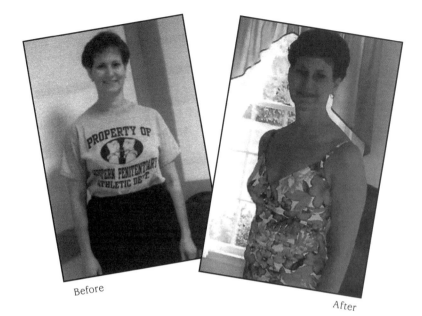

Before

After

Confession #57

Mary Beth Hassan, Camp Hill, PA
17.4 lbs. lost

I am an unconventional 53-year-old woman – unconventional in many ways. I teach convicted male felons in a state correctional institution, became water aerobics certified at 45, and I made a decision at 53 to change my lifestyle before becoming less healthy or extremely obese.

We all read stories about morbidly obese individuals who have lost extreme amounts of weight or experienced severe health issues because of unhealthy pounds. My story is less dramatic. I come from a family of emotional overeaters. I watched as my older sister grew too large to fit behind the steering wheel in her car. A younger brother, an airline captain, watched his weight and cholesterol soar following September 11th. Another brother and I fought the aging process as best we could by kicking our fitness programs into high gear.

I have been exercising on and off for 15 years. At some point during the last two years, the extra exercise that, in the past, compensated for any weight gain no longer worked. My weight gain wasn't dramatic, but it seemed to happen overnight. I blamed the weight on age, hormone replacement medication, and medical issues. My hips, back, and feet were constant sources of pain, and the extra weight gain compounded those physical problems.

A year ago, I joined a local fitness club where I noticed a brochure about a weight loss program located next door – Healthy Inspirations. One day last September, without an appointment or any planning, my curiosity about Healthy Inspirations prompted me to walk into their office. I was warmly greeted by a Healthy Inspirations staff member. After a short discussion, I wasn't sold on the idea that by simply changing my eating habits along with exercise, I could lose weight. I didn't join Healthy Inspirations that day in September, but a week later, I returned. I decided to give the Healthy Inspiration program a chance. But I informed (the staff) that my daily bagels, glasses of margaritas after a long walk, and 64-ounce water requirement were non-negotiable changes. However, once I started the Healthy Inspirations program, I gave in!

I began to lose one or two pounds a week, and the small success of that weight loss proved to be the encouragement I needed to continue making better choices about the food I consumed. Once dreading the journalizing aspect of Healthy Inspirations, I became excited to monitor my food intake and discuss my success with Healthy Inspirations' staff. I discovered the differences between proteins, starches, dairy foods, and what my body needed to maintain a healthy weight. During the past seven months, I have never missed a weekly weigh-in.

In early December, I reached my ideal weight, which is what I weighed in 1980! But I wasn't convinced that I should purchase any new clothes because I saw this weight loss as temporary. However, it is almost April and I have continued to eat healthy, exercise regularly, and maintain my ideal weight. While many women cringe about trying on bathing suits, I'm excited to see my new, toned figure in a bathing suit that is not a black, one-piece style.

With the help of Healthy Inspirations, I have made the "inside" adjustment, and my regular exercise program has provided the much needed toning and conditioning to my body. I want to continue to be a healthy, happy, physically fit woman. I recognize that I will need to make healthy choices a day at a time to maintain my healthy lifestyle. Thank you Healthy Inspirations!

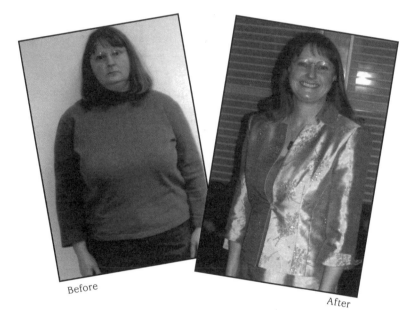

Before

After

Confession #58

Donna Schaan, Madison, WI
70 lbs. lost

This is what happened when fear started to control my life. There I was a fifty-year-old woman, whose doctor just told me that I needed to do something about my ability to absorb calcium. I would soon become one of those hunched over old ladies if I didn't turn my life around. I was too young to be this old lady and yet I did not have a clue how or where to begin this process of change.

It happened in a shopping mall parking lot, as I sadly sat questioning my life, I focused on a sign that said "Healthy Inspirations." I told myself that I supposed that I could get inspired, scary as that seemed. So in I went to meet my future. I sat down and listened while the counselor told me how I could get into an exercise program that would help me rebuild my body fitness, retrieve my daily energy as it once had been, and lose the weight…What's more it was not one of those quick fixes that six months later you ask what went wrong. I needed something for the rest of my life! Well, that was March 2005, and to date I have lost 70 pounds, over 38 inches, can easily walk miles, find each day a joy, and have my doctor thrilled with my success.

I suppose the best part of the program is that my counselors have all become my coaches and friends. They have walked me through the holidays with tips and ways for me to reach my goal. They hosted special workshops that massaged me, updated my make-up, helped me cook better tasting meals with more variety, and kept my exercise program from ever becoming boring. Just about the time I thought that is was too hard to continue, one of the counselors zipped out a tape measure and started reminding me of the bottom line or even worse showed me exactly how I looked on the day I walked through the door. They never gave up on me.

These counselors promised me many things and have lived up to every promise. They guided my meal plans, my exercise program, supported my emotional ups and downs, and best of all helped me to laugh through many of my daily woes. It doesn't get any better and they helped me to become the best me. Thank you Healthy Inspirations.

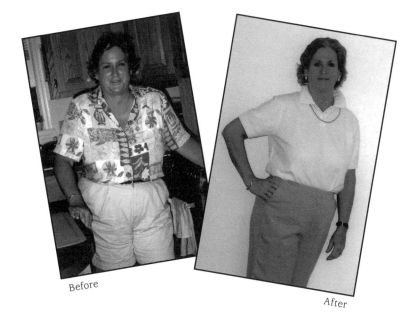

Before

After

Confession #59

Cate Meffert, Middletown, RI
40 lbs. lost

I had gone through the holidays (Thanksgiving, Christmas and
New Years) feeling terrible about myself. As much as I was looking
forward to being with family and friends at holiday festivities, I was
also dreading it! I wanted to look good and yet it was a constant
and very painful struggle to find clothes to wear that looked halfway
decent yet fit well enough to breathe! I felt horrible and was very
frustrated. Most of the time, I would rather not go than put myself
through all of that. I was basically dropping out of life, completely
beating myself up and losing every bit of self-esteem I ever had. I
was truly disgusted with myself! I have tried diets over the years,
many in fact. I would lose a few pounds here and there but nothing
substantial. Now, a few pounds were not going to cut it! Not only was
I physically uncomfortable, but I had been put on medication for
high blood pressure. I am 56 years old, have a wonderful husband,

4 children and 3 grandchildren. I want to live and live a long time to be around for all of them, but now my weight and my health could threaten all my hopes and dreams. It also was about quality of life and I was not experiencing it!

Before New Years, I began thinking about new promises and resolutions that I would make, but this time was different. I wanted it badly, very badly but was unsure of exactly how I was going to go about tackling what seemed to be a monumental challenge. Then, a friend told me about Healthy Inspirations. We shared our frustrations over weight issues, or lack of success and how awful it made each of us feel. Now, perhaps there was something or someone out there that could really help us! That was the beginning of my new life!

Basically, I showed up for my appointment with the Healthy Inspirations consultant and kept showing up. The program was explained to me in great detail. It laid out meal plans, gave "do's and don'ts" of eating, choices of foods and the amounts. All I had to do was follow it! I loved that it told me everything I needed to know right there in black and white. It also provided me with a place to go exercise as well as the incentive. God forbid, I ever really got on the floor at home myself for more than a couple of token times. It never did last! Now, I could show up at whatever time worked best for me and just play "follow the leader" around the circuit. Easy, really! That doesn't mean that it didn't take a lots of hard work and an ongoing conviction to achieve my personal goal, but that desire along with the never ending support of the program consultants have made success a reality. I feel better, look better, my blood pressure is normal and most of all I can participate in life with all of the confidence I deserve. I have lost an amazing 40 pounds and 24 inches. That truly is success. Thank you Healthy Inspirations!

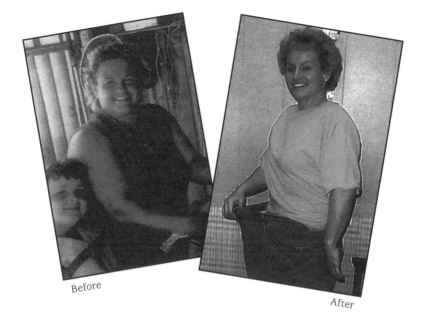

Before

After

Confession #60

Lisa Guest, Ottumwa, IA
70 lbs. lost

I was heavy and unhealthy a couple of years ago. Boy, have things changed for the better! It took all of my energy to enter the doors of a place that is now part of my daily routine. I weighed in at a hefty 206 pounds on that fall day. I was so embarrassed. That scale couldn't be right. I had gained weight after having children and working and going to school full-time. No more excuses. The time had come to improve my health and my self-esteem.

After my reality check, I volunteered and was chosen to be a participant in the Healthy Inspirations first weight-loss study in October of 2003. The results that I have achieved have been awesome! I lost 70 pounds in six months and have kept it off for over a year. I followed the program through completely. The combination of diet and exercise worked wonders for me. After I reached my goal, I then went through the balance and lifestyle phases of the program. I am in the best health and shape of my life at the age of 36.

Healthy Inspirations has given me my life back. My health has improved. I enjoy spending time with my family and friends. My outlook on life is positive. I have recently gone through an emotional time in my personal life, and the support from the staff has been truly appreciated. The advice that I would give to others is to invest in yourself. If you don't take care of your health and wellbeing, no one else will.

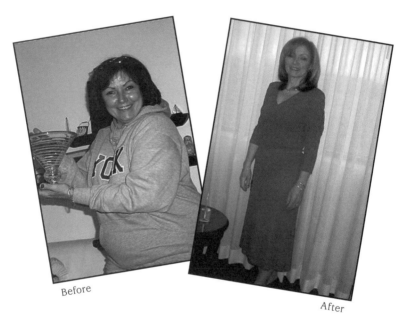

Before

After

Confession #61

Doreene Baughman, York, PA
75+ lbs. lost

Looking back, 1999 now seems a long distance away. Sometimes you have to look back to really appreciate what you have accomplished. In 1999, my dad died suddenly. My mom lived alone for about a year and because she couldn't take care of herself, her house had to be sold and she moved into an assisted living community. In 2000, my son graduated from high school and went on to college. My mother then suffered from several more strokes, which put her into a nursing facility and she ended up in the dementia unit. My best friend, supporter, and confidant was slowing fading away. She passed away in 2002.

In 2001, I was diagnosed with ankylosing spondylitis. This type of arthritis affected my lower back and hips. I was in constant pain. I went into a depression and was put on an antidepressant. After gaining even more weight, I was put on another antidepressant that did not cause weight gain. With family issues, personal issues and health issues, I felt like my life was over. I would get up, go to work, come home and lay down. I never felt more alone in my whole life. If there was a hell, I was in it.

One day my son suggested that I join Healthy Inspirations. That was in June 2005, and that was the beginning of my journey. The first couple of weeks while I was working out, I thought, "I wonder how long it will take before I fail at this." One thing I did not possess was "self-confidence". I worked out three times a week and followed a healthy eating lifestyle. With the support of the counselors at every workout and talking with the other ladies also in the program, I was encouraged, motivated, and listened to. As a result, I lost 75 plus pounds, 41 plus inches, went from a size 2X to a size 8. My depression is gone! My arthritis pain is at a minimum. I feel like a new person and I have been told I look like one too.

On March 28th, 2006, I reached my goal. It has been nine months since I started the program. In less than a year, I have turned my life around with the support of Healthy Inspirations staff, friends and family. Thank you all for your support! The program works!

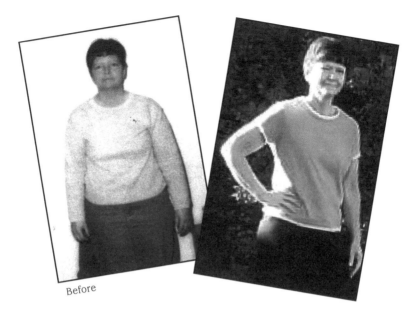

Before

Confession #62

Dianna Hubbard, Ottumwa, IA
40 lbs. lost

I joined in April 2004. I weighed 163 pounds and wore a size 14. My daughter bought me a one-week gift certificate for Valentine's Day in February 2003. I ended up misplacing it, and I found it almost a year later. I decided to call and make an appointment. I received a free week of exercise and a consultation to Healthy Inspirations. Before I really thought about it, I knew that was what I really wanted to do. I called my husband and talked it over with him and he told me to go for it.

My goal was to lose 40 pounds. When (the Lifestyle Consultant) told me I could be 123 pounds by July 2004, I couldn't believe it. I knew I was right on track. I stuck to the diet 100%. I reached my goal on schedule. I exercised at the Center five times a week and I also tried to walk with my daughter at least six or seven times a week. The staff were great. They gave me so much support. They meet with you three times a week to keep you on track. At the meetings, they weigh you and give you advice. They also help you with any problems that you may have.

Since I have lost my weight, I have much more confidence in myself. I feel so much happier and I have more energy. I no longer have problems with my feet. I often catch myself buying a lot more clothes. I actually leave the fitting rooms with a smile on my face because it is no longer a chore to try on clothes.

Now that I've reached my goal, I've changed my eating habits. I plan to keep my weight off. Once in awhile, I will eat something I really crave, but I'll get right back on track. I have tried other diets but never once was able to achieve my goal. My goal was to have my weight off for my 50th birthday and I did it. Without the program, I never would have lost the weight. My advice to others who have struggled with losing weight would be to know that you can do it. It is very hard to stick with a diet, but it is so much easier to do it with support. I am just so blessed that my daughter introduced me to the program. I would strongly suggest it to anyone because it really works!

Appendix B

BMR and the Harris-Benedict Equation

BMR Formula for Women:

BMR =   655 + (4.35 x weight in pounds) + (4.7 x height in inches)
         - (4.7 x age in years)

BMR =   655 + (4.35 x _____ lb) + (4.7 x _____ in) - (4.7 x _____)

Total = _____

Now use the Harris Benedict Equation to work out requirements including exercise:

To determine your total daily calorie needs, multiply your BMR by the appropriate activity factor, as follows:

1   If you are sedentary (little or no exercise) :
    Calorie-Calculation = BMR x 1.2
2   If you are lightly active (light exercise/sports 1-3 days/week) :
    Calorie-Calculation = BMR x 1.375
3   If you are moderately active (moderate exercise/sports 3-5 days/
    week) : Calorie-Calculation = BMR x 1.55
4   If you are very active (hard exercise/sports 6-7 days a week) :
    Calorie-Calculation = BMR x 1.725
5   If you are extra active (very hard exercise/sports & physical job
    or 2x training) : Calorie-Calculation = BMR x 1.9

Total = _____ kcal

Appendix C

Calorie Counter

Beverages	Calories
Alcoholic Beverages	**Calories**
1 oz 80 proof distilled alcohol	64
1 oz 86 proof alcohol	70
1 oz 100 proof alcohol	82
12 oz regular beer	146
12 oz light beer	99
3.5 oz red wine	74
3.5 oz rose wine	73
3.5 oz white wine	70
Carbonated Beverages	**Calories**
16 oz Club Soda	0
16 oz Cola	202
16 oz Ginger Ale	166
16 oz Diet Cola w/aspartame	5
16 oz Diet Cola w/saccharin	0
11 oz Tonic Water	114
Coffee and Tea	
8 oz coffee brewed with tap water	5
6 oz instant coffee prepared w/water	3
6 oz instant decaf coffee prepared with water	3
8 oz tea brewed w/tap water	2
8 oz herbal tea other than chamomile	2
8 oz herbal tea or chamomile	2
Fruit Juices	**Calories**
8 oz apple juice	117
8 oz apricot nectar	141

	Calories
8 oz grapefruit juice, canned, unsweetened	94
8 oz grape juice, unsweetened	154
1 oz lemon juice	8
1 oz lime juice	8
8 oz orange juice	112
8 oz pineapple juice	140
8 oz canned prune juice	182
Dairy Products	**Calories**
0.5 oz/1 Tbsp butter without salt	102
1 oz blue cheese	100
1 oz Camembert	90
1 oz Cheddar	110
1 oz Colby	110
8 oz/1 cup large curd cottage cheese	217
8 oz/1 cup dry cottage cheese	123
8 oz/1 cup cottage cheese 2% fat	203
8 oz/1 cup cottage cheese 1% fat	164
0.5 oz/1 Tbsp cream cheese	51
0.5 oz/1 Tbsp fat free cream cheese	13
1 oz Feta	75
1 oz semi soft goat cheese	103
1 oz Gouda	101
1 oz Gruyere	115
1 oz Limburger	93
1 oz Monterey	105
1 oz whole milk mozzarella	80
1 oz part skim milk mozzarella	72
1 oz Muenster	110
1 oz. Parmesan, grated	130
1 oz Provolone	100

	Calories
4.5 oz/0.5 cup whole milk Ricotta	216
4.5 oz/0.5 cup part skim milk Ricotta	180
1 oz Romano	109
1 oz Roquefort	105
1 oz Swiss	110

Milk and Cream	Calories
8 oz/1 cup whole milk	150
8 oz/1 cup 2% fat milk with vitamin A	121
8 oz/1 cup 1% fat milk with vitamin A	102
8 oz/1 cup skim milk with vitamin A	86
8 oz/1 cup buttermilk	99
8 oz/1 cup dry skim milk	434
8 oz/1 cup dry whole milk	635
8 oz/1 cup canned, condensed, sweetened milk	982
8 oz/1 cup canned evaporated skim milk	199
8 oz/1 cup goat milk	168

Cream	Calories
0.5 oz/1 Tbsp Half & Half	20
8 oz/1 cup light whipping cream	699
8 oz/1 cup heavy whipping cream	821
0.5 oz/1 Tbsp heavy whipping cream	50
8 oz/1 cup sour cream	493
0.5 oz/1 Tbsp sour cream	30

Ice Cream	Calories
4 oz/0.5 cup chocolate ice-cream	142
4 oz/0.5 cup strawberry ice-cream	127
4 oz/0.5 cup vanilla ice-cream	133
4 oz/0.5 cup vanilla ice milk	92

Yogurt	Calories
8 oz/1 cup plain whole milk yogurt	150
8 oz/1 cup plain low fat yogurt	155
8 oz/1 cup plain skim milk yogurt	137

Beans & Legumes	Calories
6 oz/1 cup cooked black beans	227
6 oz/1 cup cooked fava beans	187
6 oz/1 cup canned chick peas	286
6 oz/1 cup cooked Great Northern Beans	209
6 oz/1 cup cooked Kidney Beans	225

	Calories
16 oz/1 cup cooked lentils	230
6 oz/1 cup large cooked lima beans	216
6 oz/1 cup cooked Navy Beans	258
6 oz/1 cup cooked Peas, split	231
1 oz dry roasted peanuts	166

Beans & Legumes	Calories
1.2 oz/2 Tbsp chunky style peanut butter	188
1.2 oz/2 Tbsp smooth peanut butter	190
6 oz/1 cup cooked soy beans	298
8 oz/1 cup soy milk	81
1 Tbsp soy sauce (made from soy & wheat)	8
1 Tbsp soy sauce (made from soy)	11
1 cup tempeh	330
1 cup raw regular tofu	188
1 cup small cooked white beans	254

Fats & Oils	Calories
0.5 oz/1 Tbsp chicken fat	115
0.5 oz/1 Tbsp lard	115
0.5 oz/1 Tbsp hard margarine	34
0.5 oz/1 Tbsp soft margarine	34
0.5 oz/1 Tbsp margarine blend (60% corn oil & 40% butter)	102
0.5 oz/1 Tbsp almond oil	120
0.5 oz/1 Tbsp canola oil	124
0.5 oz/1 Tbsp corn oil	120
0.5 oz/1 Tbsp olive oil	119
0.5 oz/1 Tbsp peanut oil	119
0.5 oz/1 Tbsp sesame oil	120
0.5 oz/1 Tbsp wheat germ oil	120
0.5 oz/1 Tbsp soybean oil	120

Fruits	Calories
3 ½ inch raw apple with skin	124
1 cup dried sulfured uncooked apples	209
1 cup raw apricot halves	74
1 cup apricot halves, canned with skin	117
1 raw California avocado without skin and seeds	306
1 raw Florida avocado without skin and seeds	340
1 cup raw banana	138

1 cup raw blackberries	75
1 pint raw blueberries	225
1 cup sour red cherries	0
1 cup sweet cherries	84
1 cup European black currants	71
1 cup dried, zante currants	408
1 cup gooseberries	184
1 cup grapefruit	74
1 cup grapes, American style	58
1 cup grapes, seedless European style	114
1 large kiwi fruit without skin	56
1 kumquat without refuse	12
1 mango without refuse	135
1 cup melon balls	62
1 cup diced melon or honeydew	60
1, 2 ½ inch nectarine	67
1 large olive ripe & canned	0
1 jumbo olive ripe & canned	1
1 California navel orange	64
1 California Valencia orange	59
1 Florida orange	65
1 large tangerine	43
1 cup tangerines, canned	92
1 cup raw papaya	55
1 passion fruit	17
1 large peach	68
1 medium pear	98
1 cup diced pineapple	76
1 cup sliced plantains, cooked	179
1 plum	36
1 pomegranate	105
1 prickly pear	42
1 quince	52
1 cup seedless raisins	495
1 cup raw raspberries	60
1 cup diced rhubarb	289
1 cup raw strawberry halves	46
1 cup watermelon balls	50

Vegetables

	Calories
1 medium artichoke	60
1 small spear asparagus	3
½ cup sliced beets	74

1 cup broccoli flowerets, raw	20
½ cup brussel sprouts	30
1 cup raw cabbage	18
1 cup raw carrots	47
½ cup cooked carrots	35
1 cup raw cauliflower	25
½ cup cooked cauliflower	14
1 cup diced celery	19
½ cup cucumber slices	7
1 cup boiled eggplant	28
½ cup raw endive	4
1 cup kale	42
1 cup butter head lettuce	7
1 cup romaine lettuce	4
1 cup iceberg lettuce	7
1 cup whole raw mushrooms	24
1 cup chopped onions	60
1 cup chopped green peppers	40
1 baked potato	115
1 boiled potato	118
1 cup radish slices	20
1 cup cooked spinach	41
1 cup sliced squash, raw	16
1 cup sliced squash, cooked	38
1 large sweet potato baked	185
1 medium sweet potato, boiled	159
1 cup sliced tomatoes	38
2 medium tomatoes	66

Pasta

Pasta	Calories
1 cup elbows	197
1 cup elbows whole wheat	174
1 cup egg noodles	213
1 cup spaghetti	197
1 cup wheat spaghetti	174

Meat

Meat	Calories

Beef (3 oz portions)	Calories
brisket, flat half, lean & fat, 0" fat, braised	183
chuck, arm pot roast, lean & fat, ¼" fat, braised	282
rib, lean & fat, ¼" fat, roasted	304

bottom round, lean & fat, ¼" fat, braised 234
eye of round, lean & fat, ¼" fat, roasted 194
tenderloin, lean & fat, ½" fat, broiled 247
ground, extra-lean 143
ground, lean, broiled 231
ground, reg, broiled 143

Pork (3 oz portions)

fresh ham, whole, lean, roasted 127
loin, whole, lean, roasted 178
center Loin (chops) 172
center Rib (chops) 186
sirloin Roast 184
cured bacon, 3 medium slices 109
cured Canadian style bacon, 2 slices grilled 86

Poultry

Chicken	Calories
½ chicken light meat and skin, fried, batter	521
½ chicken light meat and skin, roasted	38
½ chicken, dark meat and skin, fried, batter	828
½ chicken, dark meat and skin, roasted	423
½ Cornish game hen, roasted	147

Turkey	Calories
turkey breast, meat and skin, roasted	1624
turkey leg, meat and skin, roasted	1136

Fish (3 oz portion)	Calories
freshwater Bass	124
striped Bass	105
bluefish	135
carp	137
catfish	129
caviar	40
Atlantic cod	89
Pacific cod	89
haddock	95
halibut	119
pickled herring	74
lox	99

wild Atlantic salmon 154
pink salmon 126
canned sardine, 1 oz 587
sea bass 105
swordfish 131
trout 127
tuna, fresh, blue fin 156
tuna, fresh, yellow fin 118

Shellfish

20 small clams 281
1 Alaskan king crab leg 129
1 cup blue crab 137
3 oz queen crab 97
3 oz lobster 83
3 oz mussel 146
6 medium oysters, raw 42
2 large scallops 66
4 large shrimp 21
3 oz squid 148

Nuts & Seeds	Calories
1 cup almonds, dried, unbalanced	559
1 cup whole kernel almonds, unbleached	970
1 cup Brazil nuts	918
1 cup cashew nuts, dry roasted	786
1 cup cashew nuts, oil roasted	748
1 oz Chinese chestnuts	67
1 oz, macadamia nuts, dried	199
1 cup, macadamia nuts, oil roasted	962
1 cup pistachio nuts	776
1 cup sunflower seeds	745
sesame seeds, 1tbsp	52
walnuts, 1 cup, black, dried	759

Breads	Calories
1 bagel, plain	157
1 cup bread crumbs	427
1 wheat dinner roll	77
1 English muffin	134
1 burger or hotdog roll	123
1 slice pumpernickel Bread	65
1 slice raisin bread	88

1 slice rye bread	83
1 slice wheat bread	65

Crackers	Calories
1 cup bite size cheese crackers	312
1 crisp bread or rye cracker	37
1 matzoh, plain	112
1 cup plain melba toast pieces	117
1 cup oyster crackers	195

Snacks/Desserts	Calories
1 oz brownie, home recipe	112
2 oz angel food cake	129
5 oz apple crisp	229
3 oz of cheesecake	256
2 oz of crumb topped coffeecake	240
1 oz devil's food w/cream filling	105
1.5 oz fruit cake	139
1 oz pound cake	117
1.3 oz sponge cake	110
2.5 oz carrot cake	239
1 oz dark chocolate	150
1 oz hard candy	106
1 oz jelly beans	104
1 oz marzipan	128
1.5 oz milk chocolate	226
1 piece butterscotch	24
4 oz gumdrops	420
1 oz chocolate covered pretzels	130
1 oz corn chips, plain	153
1 oz cheese puffs	157
1 oz potato chips	152
1 oz potato chips, sour cream and onion	150
1 oz tortilla chips	142
1 oz animal crackers	126
0.24 oz graham crackers	30
chocolate chip cookie	48
chocolate glazed donut	175
crème filled donut	307
jelly donut	189

Fast food &Restaurants	Calories

Boston Market	Calories
Barbeque Baked Beans	330
Caesar Salad Entrée	520
Chunky Chicken Salad	370
Ham & Turkey Club w/ Cheese & Sauce	890

Burger King	Calories
Biscuit w/Bacon, Egg & Cheese	510
French Toast Sticks	500
Hash Browns	240
Cheeseburger	380
Whopper Jr. w/Cheese	460

D'Angelo Sandwich Shops	Calories
Caesar Salad w/Dressing	740
BLT w/Cheese	1170
Cheeseburger Sub, large	1060
Chicken Stir Fry D'Lite Pocket	360
Meatball Sub	520
Turkey Club Pocket	400

Domino's Pizza	Calories
12 inch, medium Deep Dish Cheese, 2 slices	477
12 inch, medium, Hand Tossed Cheese, 2 slices	347
12 inch, medium, Thin Crust Cheese, 2 slices	271
1 piece cheesy bread	103

Dunkin Donuts	Calories
Blueberry Bagel	330
Everything Bagel	340
Plain Bagel	200
1 oz Light Cream Cheese	60
1 oz Garden Veggie Cream Cheese	90
1 oz Strawberry Cream Cheese	100
Blueberry Muffin	310
3 Chocolate Glazed Munchkins	180
1 Coffee Roll	180
Coffee Coolatta w/ Whole Milk	230

Coffee Coolatta w/Skim Milk	190	Jr. Bacon Cheeseburger	380
Vanilla Coolatta w/Skim Milk	200	Garden Veggie Stuffed Pita	400

McDonalds	**Calories**	**Applebee's**	**Calories**
Apple Pie	260	Asian Chicken Salad	645
Egg McMuffin	290	Blackened Chicken Salad	410
Hot Cakes	310	Chicken Fajita Quesadilla	520
Hot Fudge Sundae	340	Chicken Roma Rollup	550
6 piece Chicken McNugget	290	Garlic Chicken Pasta	530
Small French Fries	210	Lemon Chicken Pasta	530
Big Mac	560	Veggie Quesadilla	345
Grilled Chicken Deluxe	440	Whitefish w/ Mango Salsa	435

Olive Garden	**Calories**	**Chili's**	**Calories**
Capellini Pomodoro	610	Ranch Burger	1070
Chicken Giardino	550	Mushroom Swiss Burger	910
Shrimp Primavera	740	Awesome Blossom w/sauce	2880
Minestrone Soup	80	Steak Fajita	1070
		Chicken Fajita	1020
Starbucks	**Calories**	Grilled Baby Back Ribs	1130
Americano Grande	10	Boneless Buffalo Wings	1140
Cappuccino Grande w/Low Fat Milk	110	Grilled Shrimp Alfredo	1290
Drip Coffee Grande	10		
Espresso Doppio	5	**Denny's**	**Calories**
Latte Tall w/ Low Fat Milk	140	Plain French Toast	505
Mocha w/ Whip Cream Grande		Ultimate Omelet	565
Lowfat Milk	170	Belgian Waffle w/ butter and syrup	540
Biscotti Bliss Ice Cream ½ cup	240	Sirloin Steak and Eggs	620
Vanilla Mocha Chip Ice Cream, ½ cup	270	T-Bone Steak and Eggs	990
		Albacore Tuna Melt	640
Subway	**Calories**	BLT	610
Chocolate Chip M&M cookie	210	Club Sandwich	720
Sugar Cookie	230	Patty Melt	790
6 inch Subway Club	312		
6 inch Hot Meatball	419	**Long John Silvers**	**Calories**
6 inch Tuna	542	Grilled Chicken Salad	140
Roasted Chicken Salad	162	Ocean Chef Salad	130
Steak and Cheese	212	1 order Breaded Clams	250
		1 serving Popcorn Shrimp	320
Wendy's	**Calories**	Chocolate Crème Pie	280
Small Frosty	330	Strawberries N' Cream Pie	280
Baked Potato w/ Bacon and Cheese	530		
Breaded Chicken Sandwich	440		
5 piece Chicken Nugget	230		

Mrs. Fields Cookies	Calories
Chewy Fudge Cookie	220
Cinnamon Sugar Cookie	300
Debra's Special	280
Milk Chocolate Chip	280
Peanut Butter	310
Oatmeal Raisin	180
Triple Chocolate	220
Double Fudge Brownie	360

Taco Bell	Calories
Taco Supreme	260
Soft Taco Chicken	190
Double Decker Taco Supreme	420
Cheesy Gordita Crunch	560
Gordita Supreme Chicken	300
Gordita Supreme Beef	300
Chalupa Supreme Chicken	360
Chalupa Supreme Beef	380
Meximelt	290
Nachos Supreme	440
Bean Burrito	370
Chili Cheese Burrito	330
7 Layer Burrito	520

✳

Appendix D

Training Heart Rate Zone

Another way to keep an exercise program safe is to monitor your heart rate to stay within the proper training heart rate zone. Training Heart Rate (THR) means a rate at which the heart beats safely and effectively, leaving one energized after a workout, not exhausted. To determine your THR range, use the following formula, subtract your age from 220:

220- (your age) = Your maximum predicted heart rate _____

Depending upon one's age and your medical conditions, you should exercise between 60% and 80% of your Maximum Heart Rate (MHR). Not clear. To determine your THR, take your MHR calculated above and multiple that by the percentage of training desired. A 42 year old would make the calculation as follows.

220- 42 (age) = 178 MHR

178 x 0.6 (60%) = 107 minimum recommended THR, or:

178 x 0.8 (80%) = 142 maximum recommended THR.

Therefore in the example above, the THR range is between 107 and 142 beats per minute (bpm). To stay within one's THR zone, the heart rate needs to be monitored. This can be done manually but accuracy is difficult to obtain. The best and easiest way to monitor your heart rate is by investing in a heart rate monitor from a local sports store.

Appendix E

Daily Journal Page

Date: _____   Daily Caloric Limit:_____

Food or Beverage Item: # of Calories:

_____   _____

_____   _____

_____   _____

_____   _____

_____   _____

_____   _____

_____   _____

_____   _____

_____   _____

Total Daily Caloric Intake: _____

Today's
Exercise: _____

Approximate
Calories Burned:_____

**Subtract Calories burned
from Daily Caloric Intake**

*If this total is *greater* than your daily caloric limit (as recorded above), there is danger of weight gain. If this total is *less* than your daily caloric limit, weight loss success is within reach!

Appendix F

Casey Conrad

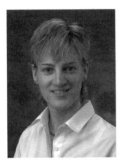

Casey Conrad has been in the health and fitness industry since 1983. She has been a featured or keynote presenter in 15 countries providing programs for communities, working in-house for companies and speaking for a variety of organizations. She is a regular featured columnist in numerous industry publications and local newspapers, has been a guest on dozens of radio talk shows and has made numerous television appearances, including the Today Tonight show in Australia.

In 1999 Ms. Conrad founded the international chain of weight loss centers called Healthy Inspirations, of which she is the President. To date there are over 70 licensed or franchised locations around the world. Ms. Conrad co-owns three Healthy Inspirations Centers that operate in Rhode Island.

She earned her BA at The American University and her JD at Roger Williams University School of Law. In addition, she is certified in Neuro-Linguistic Programming and Neuro-Associative Conditioning.

Ms. Conrad is available for speaking engagements and can be reached at 800-725-6147 or casey@healthyinspirations.us.

Appendix G

About Healthy Inspirations

Healthy Inspirations is a women's weight loss and lifestyle center focusing on long-term weight loss. With over seventy locations world-wide, Healthy Inspirations provides nutritional guidance, exercise, relaxation therapy, and personal coaching and support for its members. The Healthy Inspirations plan guarantees a weight loss of 2-3 pounds per week. Members receive encouragement and motivation to not only achieve their weight loss goals, but to maintain a healthy weight for life. For more information on the Healthy Inspirations program or franchising opportunities in the United States, visit www.healthyinspirations.us or call 1-800-725-6147, and in Australia, visit www.healthyinspirations.com.au or call 1300-LOSE WEIGHT.